ORGANISATIONAL INNOVATION IN HEALTH SERVICES

Lessons from the NHS treatment centres

John Gabbay, Andrée le May, Catherine Pope, Glenn Robert

With Paul Bate and Mary-Ann Elston

'N

D0574238

First published in Great Britain in 2011 by

The Policy Press
University of Bristol
Fourth Floor
Beacon House
Queen's Road
Bristol BS8 1QU
UK

t: +44 (0)117 331 4054
f: +44 (0)117 331 4093
tpp-info@bristol.ac.uk
www.policypress.co.uk

North American office:
The Policy Press
c/o International Specialized Books Services
920 NE 58th Avenue, Suite 300
Portland, OR 97213-3786, USA
t: +1 503 287 3093
f: +1 503 280 8832
info@isbs.com

© The Policy Press 2011

British Library Cataloguing in Publication Data
A catalogue record for this book is available from the British Library.

Library of Congress Cataloging-in-Publication Data
A catalog record for this book has been requested.

ISBN 978 1 84742 478 5 paperback
ISBN 978 1 84742 479 2 hardcover

The right of John Gabbay, Andrée le May, Catherine Pope, Glenn Robert with Paul Bate and Mary-Ann Elston to be identified as authors of this work has been asserted by them in accordance with the Copyright, Designs and Patents Act 1988.

Cover design by The Policy Press.
Front cover: image kindly supplied by Elliott Pope.
Printed and bound in Great Britain by TJ International, Padstow.
The Policy Press uses environmentally responsible print partners.

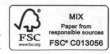

To those who, at every level of all health services, are trying ceaselessly to improve their organisations.

Contents

List of abbreviations

A&E	accident and emergency (department)
ACAD	Ambulatory Care and Diagnostic Centre
DH	Department of Health ('the Department')
DTC	diagnosis and treatment centre
GP	general practitioner
G–Supp	General Supplementary (payment)
NHS	National Health Service
NIHR	National Institute for Health Research
PCT	primary care trust
PFI	private finance initiative
SDO	Service Delivery and Organisation (an NIHR research programme)
SHA	strategic health authority
TC	treatment centre

Notes on the authors

John Gabbay is Emeritus Professor, Wessex Institute for Health Research and Development, University of Southampton. From 1992–2004, as Professor of Public Health in Southampton, he directed the Wessex Institute for Health Research and Development and the National Co-ordinating Centre for Health Technology Assessment. Since qualifying in Medicine at Manchester in 1974, he has published over 100 papers across subjects ranging from the social history of medicine, through public health to NHS management, but his main focus has been the social and organisational origins of medical knowledge. His recent work has concentrated on the way that knowledge enters policy and practice.

He participated in designing the research, carried out the fieldwork at one site, helped analyse the findings and took the lead in writing the final research report and this book.

Andrée le May was Professor of Nursing in the School of Health Sciences, University of Southampton until her partial retirement. Known internationally for her work on the development of evidence-based practice in nursing, she has published extensively on the dissemination and implementation of research. She was responsible for developing and running one of the leading clinical doctorate programmes in the UK and has run many courses on healthcare leadership. Her recent work has focused on the role of communities of practice in the spread of knowledge and innovation in health services.

She participated in designing the research, carried out fieldwork at one site and participated in the analysis and in the writing of the research report and this book.

Catherine Pope is Professor of Medical Sociology, Faculty of Health Sciences, University of Southampton. She is widely known for her proselytising work on qualitative methods in health services research. Her many publications include seminal evaluations of the processes of healthcare organisation and delivery, notably studies of waiting lists, advanced access to general practice care and NHS Walk-in Centres. She has also undertaken important ethnographic studies of healthcare work and the nature of professional expertise, focusing on surgery and anaesthetic practice. She was joint editor of *Sociology*, a leading journal of the British Sociological Association. She helped develop the research design, carried out fieldwork at two sites, helped analyse the findings and contributed to the writing of the report and this book.

Glenn Robert is Senior Research Fellow, King's College London, University of London. Over the last 14 years of conducting organisational studies focusing on quality and service improvement in healthcare and new perspectives on large-scale change, he has – among many other publications – co-authored/edited four books, one of which explored how innovations in healthcare delivery and organisation spread, which won the 2006 Baxter Award for the most outstanding contribution to healthcare management in Europe.

He jointly had the idea for the study, participated in designing the research, led the sampling, carried out fieldwork at three sites and participated in the analysis of the findings and in the writing. He took the lead in drafting the material in the original research report that now comprises Chapter Four and also the joint lead (with Paul Bate) for what are now Chapters Seven and Eight of this book.

Paul Bate, Professor Emeritus, Royal Free and University College Medical School, London, has published extensively in the international literature and written several books on organisational development and change management, healthcare research, policy and practice. He was closely involved in the modernisation and reform of the NHS following the publication of The NHS Plan in 2000, working with governmental and other agencies.

He jointly had the idea for the study, participated in designing the research, carried out fieldwork at one site, helped analyse the findings, participated in writing the report, where he took the joint lead (with Glenn Robert) in drafting the final chapter on which the current Chapters Seven and Eight are based. Having retired in the interim, he took no further part in the writing of this book.

Mary Ann Elston is Emeritus Reader in Medical Sociology, Royal Holloway, University of London and Visiting Reader in Sociology at the University of Surrey. She spent 30 years as a researcher and teacher in medical sociology, mainly at Royal Holloway, where she was Director of the MSc in Medical Sociology from 1993 to 2003. Her main areas of research are in the sociology and social history of healthcare occupations and organisations, gender in the medical profession and medical careers, and social movements and health. From 1994 to 2000 she was joint editor of the international journal, *Sociology of Health and Illness*.

She carried out the literature review that formed the basis of Chapter One and participated in the writing of the book.

Introduction

Those who ignore the lessons of history are condemned to repeat it. (George Santayana)

Learning from case studies of an NHS innovation

When the UK government announced in 2000 that over 40 major diagnosis and treatment centres (DTCs) would be introduced across the National Health Service (NHS), the idea was generally acclaimed as one whose time had come. DTCs were an innovative way of providing healthcare to thousands of patients with specific healthcare needs (see Appendix 1). Mostly purpose-built, DTCs would be designed to ensure that elective patients requiring straightforward diagnosis or treatment would avoid long waits and unnecessary hospital stays. DTCs would, moreover, spearhead the modernisation of ways of working in the NHS, another equally important priority that included the redefinition of professional roles and the spread of pre-defined pathways of patient care. Hospitals throughout the NHS rushed to get involved. Within a year of the original announcement, eight DTCs were already up and running, and by the end of 2006 there were 46 in place, with many more being planned. Yet, as with so many healthcare innovations, these DTCs or treatment centres (TCs), as they were later relabelled, did not turn out quite as central government had originally envisaged.

Although TCs are now an established part of the NHS, the lessons that we learned from studying their introduction remain poignantly relevant, since similar large-scale initiatives in the organisation and delivery of healthcare are – and are always likely to be – a continuing feature of central government policy making. There are many important questions one could ask specifically about TCs, such as whether the policy to establish them has been successful, how the new arrangements have affected patient experience and outcomes, whether professional roles changed for the better, what works or does not work in the management of elective patients and whether private sector involvement has improved the service. This book, however, focuses on a broader question – how local managers implement an innovation driven by national policy. That generic question will always retain far-reaching relevance since the tension between centrally driven, top-down policy and the local management of change is a permanent part not just of the NHS but any large healthcare system – indeed of any large public sector service in any country. And it is nearly always problematic.

This book tells the stories of eight TCs that we studied closely as they evolved from 2003-06. Their stories graphically illustrate the way in which planned innovation from on high can be transformed into a multiplicity of local solutions to different problems. The outcome was not as any policy makers or NHS staff predicted or originally intended, and this was partly because those very same policy makers were also making so many other, often conflicting, demands on the local managers and clinicians. The unfolding accounts make salutary reading.

How the book came about

Studies of major innovations in healthcare organisations have seldom been able to evaluate their growth and development over time. Greenhalgh et al (2005, p 17) argue that:

> ... the main gap in the research literature on complex service innovations in health care organisations is an understanding of how they arise, especially since this process is largely decentralised, informal and hidden from official scrutiny. An additional key question is how such innovations are reinvented as they diffuse within and between organisations.

NHS TCs presented a remarkable chance to help fill that gap by following the development of a high profile and complex public sector innovation from initial conception through its early implementation and subsequent evolution. We decided, therefore, to focus on TCs that were within the NHS, and not, except insofar as their development cut across that of the NHS TCs, on the different (and more politically controversial) parallel promotion of privately run independent sector TCs, which emerged during the course of our fieldwork. Nor do we report here a linked study in which colleagues undertook mathematical modelling designed to test assumptions about capacity requirements (such as how many beds would be needed and how patient flows might be optimised) and to identify circumstances where the introduction of a TC might (or, as it sometimes turned out, might not) improve its local health economy (Gallivan and Utley, 2005; Utley and Gallivan 2004; Utley et al, 2005, 2008, 2009). The story here is a more general and more generalisable one: what really happened on the ground as an array of social, political, institutional, cultural and economic factors impacted on a major national programme of health service innovation that involved various professional groups as well as major technological and organisational change.

Our fieldwork was based on over 200 interviews with key stakeholders in the TCs, their host hospitals and their local health economies (that is, neighbouring hospital trusts,[1] community trusts and healthcare commissioners), and members of organisations whose role was to help the development of the TC programme. We also observed TC staff in action (including training sessions, planning and management meetings, general interactions between the people involved in setting up and running the TCs, the processes of care and the physical environment of the TCs) and scrutinised documents including business plans, hospital governance documents and marketing materials. (For further methodological details see Appendix 2.) Our findings appeared in a long and detailed research report to the funders of the study, the National Institute for Health Research Service Delivery and Organisation (NIHR SDO) Programme. We also decided, however, to write this much shorter book because it seemed to us that the story was relevant not just to academics and students of organisational sciences who might be willing to download and read a 280-page research report (Bate et al, 2006), but would also be of interest to established and trainee health service managers, policy makers, planners and practitioners who are having to deal in their everyday work with organisational innovations and change management challenges of this type. These are the very people who may find it helpful to read a brief independent account of a world that is familiar to them, but one that is often bewildering and rarely discussed explicitly. It is for them that we have tried here to present the findings, link them to relevant lessons from the wider field of organisational studies and spell out the practical lessons in a relatively short and readable form. We hope that our analysis of this piece of very recent NHS history may help readers to make sense of future major organisational innovations in health services, and perhaps help them to prepare for some of the challenges they are likely to face.

Outline

Chapter One is based on our review of the literature and outlines the origins of the TC model, based largely on the US ambulatory care model that preceded the launch of the UK government's TC programme. We explore the background to that programme, including the reasons behind the initiative and the intentions that the government and Department of Health had for it when they launched it in *The NHS Plan* (DH, 2000a). We also briefly outline

–

the subsequent rapid development of the programme and the part played by the Modernisation Agency, an organisation that had been set up to facilitate and oversee the 'modernising' programmes that the government envisaged. Chapter Two describes the internal and external milieux of all eight sites, which formed the context for the organisational innovation we were studying. We show how varied the local cultures and concerns were that lay behind the decision to open a TC as part of the national programme, and we describe what we call the opportunists, idealists, pragmatists and sceptics who were engaged in the debates about that decision. In Chapter Three we thematically analyse the motivating factors that persuaded the senior teams in the eight sites to establish a TC in their locality, grouped into the main categories of the desire to improve: (1) quality, such as redesigned patient pathways; (2) quantity, such as patient throughput; and (3) kudos, including both organisational and individual profile and status. The main government and Department of Health policy initiatives that subsequently affected the TCs, such as the increasing emphasis and encouragement given to independent sector TCs, 'Patient Choice' and 'Payment by Results' schemes, are set out in Chapter Four, which also outlines the development of an organisation of a small group of TCs called 'NHS Elect' that was set up as a collective attempt to deal with the practical difficulties caused by that policy environment. In Chapters Five and Six we describe and thematically analyse how the eight TCs evolved and met their varied fates. Chapter Five discusses the ways in which initial plans rarely worked out as intended, and considers the impact played by the pressurised nature of the initial planning, by the subsequent impact of shifts in national policy, by the state of relationships with partner organisations including the host hospital, and by the internal developments and staff changes. Chapter Six describes changes to the way patient care was delivered, and discusses briefly both how these were implemented and perceived. We conclude with a summary in Chapter Seven of our main findings interpreted in the light of the literature relevant to organisational innovation, followed by Chapter Eight, where we discuss the practical implications for innovations in service delivery more generally in the NHS and other health systems.

Acknowledgements

We thank our funders, the NIHR SDO Programme, and the very constructive peer reviewers of our original research report. (The views and opinions expressed in the book are of course our own and do not necessarily reflect those of the NIHR SDO Programme or the Department of Health.) Like many of the TCs themselves, we were given a flying start in our understanding of the field by the generous help that we received from the staff of the Central Middlesex Hospital Ambulatory Care and Diagnosis Centre (ACAD), especially Sir Graham Morgan and Amanda Layton, and from the staff of the Modernisation Agency, especially Helen Bevan. We are also grateful to our colleagues from the University of London Clinical Operational Research Unit who participated in our research meetings while conducting linked operational research on TCs and whose insights were invaluable. Above all we thank the participants at our research sites for the openness with which they let us into their developing stories, and for the inspiring but salutary example they set to anyone wishing to introduce major innovations into an organisation as complex as the NHS.

It is always problematic to write an account of this sort while holding to one's assurance to the participants in the original research that the data would be kept anonymous and unattributable. We have endeavoured as best we can to keep to that promise and have therefore deliberately kept the details of most of the sites fairly vague (such matters as numbers, sizes, budgets, architecture, job titles and so on) and reported sites in such a way as to try and disguise them. However, it is inevitable that a few of those who were close to the TC programme may still be able to identify the sites. We apologise if that be the case and can only suggest that anyone who is able to do so will be 'part of the family' and already well aware of most of the matters we raise. Had we rendered the data even more anonymous the stories would have become too indistinct for readers to be able reliably to learn from what happened. Our aim in producing this book is, after all, to help policy makers and managers build on the successes and avoid the mistakes of the recent past.

Note

[1] A 'trust' is an NHS organisation that provides NHS services in England and Wales. Acting as a public sector corporation, it can be, for example, an acute (or hospital) trust that manages one or more hospitals, or it can be a community care trust a or primary care trust (PCT). During the period covered by this study, PCTs were also responsible for commissioning services for their local population from, for example, hospital, community care or mental health trusts. The commissioning and other work of the PCTs was coordinated by strategic health authorities (SHAs) or by regional offices of the Department of Health, often loosely referred to as 'the regions'.

ONE

Transplanted roots: where the innovation came from

The NHS archetype of treatment centres

'... the revolution in care that you have pioneered here is to be applied all over the country.' (former Prime Minister Tony Blair in a speech at the Ambulatory Care and Diagnostic Centre [ACAD], Central Middlesex Hospital, London, February 2001)

In a traditional hospital, the patient is certainly central to diagnostic and therapeutic preoccupations, but not to the organization. Indeed, the physician and the nursing staff are at the centre of the organisation.... The order of organisational priorities is reversed in an ambulatory surgery unit. This substantive organisational revolution is even more: it is indeed a genuine cultural revolution. (De Lathouwer, 1999)

The ACAD ... is ... a building capable of doing the work of a DGH [district general hospital] two to three times larger. (Black, 1999, p 4)

The concept of the treatment centre (TC) had roots that existed well before the 2000 *NHS Plan* that promulgated the scheme. The model of ambulatory surgical centres and other forms of 'focused factories' (Casalino and Robinson, 2003; Casalino et al, 2004), which had existed in US healthcare since the 1970s, had meant that neither the archetype nor its context was wholly new to the NHS. Indeed five planned ambulatory care centres in England, two of which subsequently became part of the TC programme, were discussed in a report in the mid-1990s (NHS Estates, 1996, p 4). But it was the Ambulatory Care and Diagnostic Centre (ACAD) opened at the Central Middlesex Hospital in North West London in 1999 that was most cited as the prototype for the TC programme.

The ACAD is a purpose-built two-storey free-standing unit on the site of, but administratively distinct from, its host hospital. The building itself won high praise and awards from architects and others involved with healthcare construction and facilities provision, which probably contributed to the ACAD's high profile in the NHS. However, the ACAD's main claim to fame was the process by which it managed a wide range of elective day case work with in-patient stays that exceeded one day in only five per cent of patients. Its distinguishing features relative to conventional day case units were the 'strong emphasis on protocol-driven care' and the significant role played by the 'scheduler' in the organisation (Bowers et al, 2002, p 306). Schedulers worked in teams directly responsible to the ACAD's manager, not to individual consultants, and their role was to make appointments according to protocols for specific procedures by liaising with patients and/or general practitioners (GPs) directly to reduce non-attendance (Morgan and Layton, 1999). These schedules had been arrived at after a detailed exercise of 'process mapping' for 126 different kinds of elective procedure, which had begun in 1994. The team at Central Middlesex Hospital – ignoring traditional organisational constraints and staff-oriented approaches – had developed integrated care pathways from first principles that focused primarily on the needs of the patients (G. Morgan and A. Layton, personal communication). This entailed a determination to redesign professional roles irrespective of traditional professional boundaries, which therefore also gave rise to a complete redesign of the skill mix and roles of ACAD clinicians. For example, nurses rotated weekly through the different activities in the centre and were graded for the purposes of payment and job responsibility not according to the conventional grades, but into three bands according to the level of multi-skill competence reached; and almost all of the many doctors who did sessional work in the ACAD were consultant grade, with only a few junior doctors. The result was a 'combination of predictable, routine patients and a reliable supply of resources [that was] to enable the delivery of streamlined health care with few sources of delay' (Bowers et al, 2002, p 308). The model of 'ambulatory care' adopted at the ACAD was based not just on the clear separation of elective and emergency cases, but also on handling only those elective patients whose requirements for diagnostic or treatment interventions and whose suitability for day or short-stay procedures had been formulated as pre-determined pathways. Moreover these pathways were literally built into the ACAD's architecture, which had been designed to allow patients to move through the building as they moved smoothly through their pre-programmed care procedures.

None of this was achieved without considerable internal political manoeuvring within the host hospital, often in the face of strong opposition from sections of the consultant body. It took a strong management team, including some influential clinicians and academics, to achieve such major changes. Their success was helped by the threat of the Central Middlesex Hospital's extinction unless something drastic was done to give it a unique edge; by a visionary desire – based on a local history of strong interest in 'patient-focused care' (linked to a US organisation) – to radically alter medical and surgical care; by the expectation that the new unit would improve patient flows while reducing costs; and by the undeniable need to upgrade poor premises and facilities.

During the period in which the ACAD was subsequently being heralded as the prototype for TCs, there was no firm published evidence as to the clinical benefits, patient satisfaction, cost reduction or cost-effectiveness at the ACAD compared to a conventional day surgery unit, five-day ward or elective inpatient surgery.[1] Sillince et al (2002, p 1428) suggest that the claims of 40 per cent predicted savings which 'did much to motivate Cabinet interest' at government level may have been exaggerated as part of managerial strategy to convince opponents of the need for change. One factor that may have affected the achievement of financial forecasts is that the original business plans for the ACAD assumed a competitive internal market, with the ACAD attracting referrals from many, widely spread sources. However, the change of political climate under New Labour, which initially played down the internal market, meant that referrals were mainly local (NHS Estates, 2001, p 62). The nearest thing to a published independent evaluation was produced by the NHS Estates Department and was generally very positive despite a long list of concerns about the 'teething problems' and an admission that evidence about the costs and benefits of the new service was lacking because the unit was not yet fully operational and it was too soon to have gathered relevant data. Despite this, the conclusion of this evaluation was that the ACAD had achieved a great deal, and 'must be deemed a success' (NHS Estates, 2001, p 81). Nevertheless the report urged planners to await 'incontrovertible evidence' of its providing an effective service.

They didn't. Even as that report was being written, the ACAD was already being paraded by the government and the Department of Health as an iconic innovation that could be used to legitimise radical changes in service delivery elsewhere. As far as we can ascertain, once the ACAD became fully operational no objective independent evidence of its benefits was ever published. Hence, while no one would deny that there were benefits from the redesigned services of the ACAD, objective evidence of these benefits never emerged. (It is worth noting, of course, that decisions to implement new policies and practice without formal and timely evaluation – or without attention being paid to the results of such evaluations – are not untypical in the NHS; see Sanderson, 2002; Bate and Robert, 2003.) The ACAD meanwhile, despite facing many of the problems that were to beset our sample TCs, maintained its pioneering role in ambulatory care. To this day it employs specially trained multi-skilled staff who manage all of its patients according to pre-programmed protocols that have continued to be developed since the early days.

The US ambulatory care model

Identifying the desired outcomes and core processes that implement and facilitate those outcomes is critical. Concentration on these has true value from the perspective of the patient, the physician and the investor. This process, if implemented fully, affects everything from the architectural design of the whole building to the design of an individual operating room and the operational processes necessary to provide services. (Steffes, 1999, p 2)

I can do more cases in a shorter amount of time, which means I can make more money and get finished sooner. (senior US orthopaedic surgeon, quoted in Jackson, 2002)

… as policy makers in successive British governments have discovered, it is possible to cherry pick initiatives from the US healthcare system in a pragmatic and often incremental fashion. Changing values in British society have assisted in this process by creating a context that is more receptive to the transfer of American experience. (Ham, 2005, p 598)

The model for TCs had grown from deep roots in the US, although only occasionally was that explicitly referred to. Ambulatory care of a similar mould that may also have been a partial influence could also be found in other industrialised countries, including Australia, Western Europe and perhaps the polyclinics of Eastern Europe, but these were much less clear. The US influence was often directly through visits and links with US centers, or by TCs indirectly by using the ACAD as the basis for their design which itself was at least partly inspired by the US model.

There have always been profound differences between the hospital system in the US and the NHS in England, yet 'selective borrowing' of ideas and examples of innovation from the US has been increasingly influential in NHS policy since the 1980s (Ham, 2005). Because some of the key themes in the US, such as hospital diversification and the decentralisation of services (Stoeckle, 1995, p 13), were being followed in the government's modernisation programme for the NHS, including the TC programme, we must dwell briefly also on the US model. We do this partly to highlight the extent to which policy makers borrowed selectively from the US trends when developing the NHS TC initiative, and partly to stress that although there are obvious commonalities with the UK, there are also marked differences.

By the turn of the millennium, pressure in most developed countries for cost containment, particularly of hospital expenditure, and for services to be more responsive to consumers' demands, had led to:

- a general trend of reducing the length of hospital in-patient stay;
- a growing trend towards day surgery, with new techniques such as endoscopic ('keyhole') surgery as well as new organisational arrangements;
- a shift of service delivery away from in-patient hospital services to out-patients or ambulatory-based delivery with greater input by primary and community care services;
- providers' and policy makers' interest in reorganising healthcare in ways that sought to increase efficiency and manage risk through formal protocols and guidelines even if that meant breaking with established professional and specialty demarcations;
- providers' and policy makers' interest in financial management tools, such as prospective payment systems, and in increased competition between care providers as a means of controlling cost and raising quality.

The pace and form of these changes had varied considerably between countries and the extent to which different health services developed new ways of delivering care that could be transplanted between them depended, as always, on many specific contextual features. However, by 2001, many in the UK were attracted by the US model of free-standing ambulatory surgery centres, which had been long established in the US for a number of reasons. First, their rise had been largely in competition with the traditional hospital as part of a general assault on the 'citadel' of the hospital that many commentators described as having been in crisis since the 1970s. Second, initiatives in ambulatory surgery had already begun to have an impact on the pattern of surgical services in the US by the late 1960s, so that when the most widely cited pioneering ambulatory centre, the Phoenix Surgicenter in Arizona, was opened in 1970 it was followed by widespread exponential spread over two decades. (This was very different from the sudden explosion of such centres following the central TC initiative in the UK in 2002, when the US expansion had already run its course.) Third, the ownership and motivation for US surgicenters differed from UK TCs in important respects. Most surgicenters were owned by medical practitioners who established them partly as a means of solving some of their own frustrations about their professional lives, for example by reducing on-call duties and by providing suitable facilities for 'performing ambulatory surgery under general anaesthesia not in a hospital setting and yet in a safe environment, thereby producing a revolution in health care' (Reed and Kershner, 1993, p 18). Doctors ran most of the US surgicenters to manage elective operating schedules to ensure more predictable working hours, to defend professional autonomy – particularly in the face of managed care regimes and corporatisation – and to generate income (Pham et al, 2004). Fourth, the growth of surgicenters was associated with direct consumer demand for day surgery as well as federal government and third party cost containment policies where there was overt cost-based competition between the different forms of healthcare provision. To patients and insurance companies and other third party payers, surgicenters offered cheaper facilities than in-patient hospital wards and hence had advantages for corporate investors in for-profit healthcare, especially when they were touted as investment opportunities that were exempt from state and federal attempts to limit hospital expansion. Such considerations, like many of the features in the way the centers were consequently financed and organised, were – as we shall see – very different from the UK's NHS TCs.

Surgicenters had been successful in the US, in the sense that their numbers (see Figure 1.1) and the volume of services that they provide had grown rapidly, but how they worked, and how their quality and performance might compare with alternative ways of doing the same work, were not easy to establish from the published literature. Moreover stand-alone surgical facilities were by no means uncontroversial within the US, although what evidence there was (not very robust or extensive, and not generally adjusted for risk) suggested that the overall quality and outcomes were as good if not better in these specialist facilities (Casalino and Robinson, 2003). Their contribution to the overall pattern of care in the US was relatively small, and at that stage remained contentious. Despite that, and the fact that there was almost no formal independent evaluation of the clinical or cost-effectiveness of US ambulatory care and certainly none that allows them to be applied with confidence in the UK, the ideas were without doubt 'selectively borrowed' (Ham, 2005). Certain of their key characteristics, such as patient selection according to strict protocols, the separation of elective and emergency care and an emphasis on reduced costs and patient convenience, inspired the ACAD and sowed the seeds of the NHS TC programme.

Figure 1.1: Growth of surgicenters in the US, 1971-91

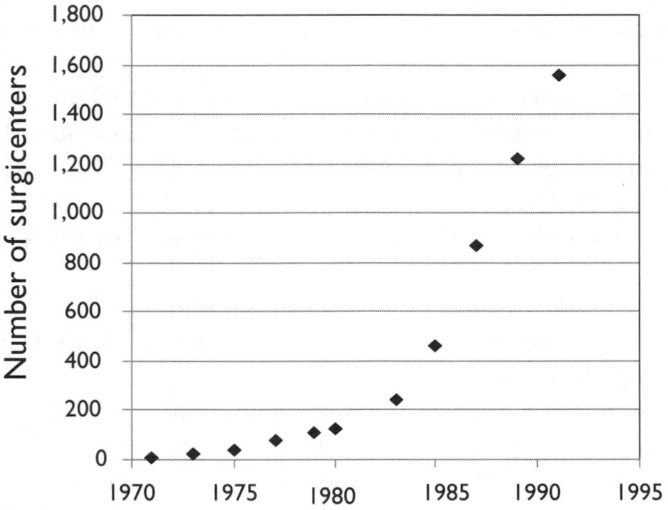

Sources: Durant (1993); Durant and Battaglia (1993)

Treatment centres and *The NHS Plan*

In partnership with the private sector we will develop a new generation of Diagnostic [sic][2] and Treatment Centres to increase the number of elective operations which can be treated on a single day or with a short stay. These Centres will separate routine hospital surgery from hospital emergency work so they can concentrate on getting waiting times down. As a result of this *NHS Plan* there will be 20 diagnostic and treatment centres developed by 2004. By then, 8 will be fully operational treating approximately 200,000 patients a year. (DH, 2000a, p 44)

Despite the growing interest in such facilities, there had been no references to diagnosis and treatment centres (DTCs) in national policy documents before *The NHS Plan* became the launch pad to develop them. With promises of major capital investment, organisational reform of the NHS and a continuing increase in the proportion of surgery undertaken as day cases, *The NHS Plan* announced that 'special one-stop diagnosis and treatment centres will concentrate on performing operations, not coping with emergencies' (DH, 2000a, p 19). The specificity of *The NHS Plan* and the four-year timescale for new capital projects to be operational suggests, as is the way with most White Papers, that the new policy initiative was in reality already under development before its official announcement, making at least some targets easy to reach. In fact the initial target was to be rapidly exceeded, such that 29 TCs had been opened (if not working fully) by mid-2004 and some 80 more, including NHS and independent sector-run TCs, were forecast by the end of 2005 (DH, 2004).

There was much else in *The NHS Plan* of relevance to the TC initiative:

- A major policy aim was to wage 'war on waiting', with TCs spearheading the attack.
- The document was replete with references to the need for organisational transformation of 'a 1940s system operating in a 21st century world' (DH, 2000a, p 15). There were 325 instances of the word 'new', 70 of 'reform', 12 of 'radical' and five of 'transformation', which set a tone of modernisation and innovation into which the TC programme fitted very clearly. References to redesigning services 'around the convenience and concerns of the patient' (DH, 2000a, p 15), to revising and reducing the boundaries between primary and secondary care, reconfiguration of workforce roles and to establishing a Modernisation Agency (to be discussed later in this chapter) to support redesign of care around patients (DH, 2005a, pp 59-60) were employing the language of radical change through 'process-based organizational transformation' (McNulty and Ferlie, 2002).[3]
- It presaged the increased involvement of the private sector in both financing capital expenditure within the NHS and in supplying healthcare for NHS patients. The development of independent sector TCs fitted within a broader and politically controversial policy framework of new partnerships between the public and private sectors in providing healthcare.
- Workforce redesign was a crucial part of the plan, which included hospital care as more of a 'consultant delivered service' (DH, 2000a,

p 78), extended roles for nurses and greater use of protocols, with specific mention of the pioneering work in this regard of the ACAD (DH, 2000a, p 83).

Reducing waiting times and more

At the Department of Health TCs rapidly became embedded among several initiatives that together represented the 'radical rethinking' required to deliver the government's waiting list targets for 2005 and 2008 (NHS Modernisation Agency, 2003b) while making care more 'patient-centred'. Thus the TC programme was set within the Department of Health's Waiting, Booking, Choice Programme whose role was 'to bring about the reforms needed to ensure NHS patients get fast and convenient access to services' (NHS Modernisation Agency, 2003a, p 2), together with the national implementation of planned booking of appointments (see Ham et al 2003), and, later, the initiation of the Patient Choice initiative[4] (DH, 2003a). The inability of the NHS itself to expand capacity sufficiently to meet the 2005 and 2008 targets and to deal with bottlenecks was the prime justification given in public for turning to the independent healthcare sector to develop additional TCs (to be discussed later) in order to 'make a real impact in time for delivering the waiting time targets in 2005 and beyond', as well as to 'lead the way in innovation, productivity and speedy response' (DH, 2002c).

In press releases, public relations and policy documents the TC programme was overwhelmingly framed in terms of reducing the wait for treatment, but the Department of Health simultaneously saw TCs as a driving force in the 'modernisation' process. TCs were intended to blaze a trail for reforms based on a restructuring of hospital care that had been discussed since the 1980s. The separation of elective from emergency surgery, the encouragement of day case or very short-stay surgery, the use of planned booking and pre-assessment clinics and the changes to skill mix and conventional divisions of labour that form the archetypal description of a TC were all orientated to faster and more predictable throughput of cases. For example, the programme was identified as contributing specifically to the Patient Choice initiative and to other NHS targets such as reduction in out-patient waiting, increased day surgery rates, reduction in cancelled operations, improving emergency care access and improving the patient experience (Thompson, 2003). Policy makers also recognised the potential of the TC programme, particularly with respect to the envisaged role of the independent sector, for increasing competitive pressures on conventional NHS elective care delivery. Finally, the modernisation theme embedded in the TC programme, and especially the call for workforce restructuring, had more than a whiff of the potential to undermine the sometimes politically unpopular autonomy of the medical profession.

Development of the treatment centres programme 2000-04

Progress was rapid by NHS standards, with more than twice the number of centres being at least partly operational by 2004 than had been proposed in 2000.[5] All eight of the first wave TCs opened their doors on time (NHS Modernisation Agency, 2003b). However, progress was not, apparently, rapid enough for the government to be confident of reaching its waiting list targets by the General Election in 2005. In *The NHS Plan*, the involvement of the private sector in TC development had been flagged as a non-specific possibility; for example, it was merely assumed that many NHS TCs might involve some private financing, a controversial theme that the government was increasingly advocating in policy-making circles. But two years later in 2002 came the explicit initiative to involve the independent sector as direct providers of TC clinical services, with the clear expectation that, in the words of the head of the implementation team responsible for this development, these independent sector TCs, would have 'shorter set up times than the NHS is used to' (Architects for Health, 2003). From 2002, the NHS-run and independent sector TC-run programmes were pursued in parallel[6] (see Chapter Four).

Role of the Modernisation Agency

Following *The NHS Plan*, the Department of Health established an NHS Modernisation Agency to promote service development, largely by spreading 'know-how' about best practice. The agency had a specific (D)TC team which developed extensive guidance, ran seminars and training events and provided advice and help to local initiatives, offering that '[a]s soon as a new DTC is confirmed, a member of the MA [Modernisation Agency] DTC team will get in touch to offer as much support and guidance as is requested' (NHS Modernisation Agency, 2003a, p 6). The agency's team produced an online 'Step guide' for those considering setting up TCs, and its website contained information about the national programme and some individual TCs as well as a number of publications specifically on TCs. These included a newsletter, *Cutting*

Edge, aimed at those working in or developing TCs, an overview of TCs as a new service model and a report on lessons from the first wave TC sites, based on interviews with key informants (NHS Modernisation Agency, 2003a, 2003b). Thus the Modernisation Agency offered itself as a major source of advice and coordination, conveying lessons for the early pioneering sites. These early lessons included:

- the need to ring-fence TCs so that emergency demands did not encroach;
- the importance of planning and the long time needed to get an operational plan together;
- the huge effort that would be involved in, for example, redesigning patient pathways and refurbishing existing buildings;
- the likely problems and advantages of detailed workforce planning;
- the need for advanced project management skills and careful risk management;
- the dangers of being rushed to get the TC up and running without robust preparation;
- the need to engage with all the likely stakeholders through a comprehensive communications strategy; and
- the value of learning from other TCs, preferably via the agency itself.

The agency did indeed play a vital role in putting the Department of Health's policy into practice and leading the early development of TCs.[7] But the breakneck speed at which the programme developed was a function of the way in which local hospitals and associated healthcare organisations jumped at the scheme, and it is to those local circumstances that we now turn, beginning with a look at the pre-existing conditions that were to shape our sample of eight TCs.

Notes

[1] Since the 1980s day surgery units had been increasingly introduced into the NHS as had five-day and short-stay wards for elective patients, but the ACAD had taken this trend a step further by re-engineering a more streamlined process for such patients, which entailed radical restructuring of staff, the processes of care and the environment.

[2] It is worth noting this reference to what it then called diagnostic and treatment centres. The correct original term was 'diagnosis and treatment centres'. Shortly after the arrival of a new Secretary of State for Health in 2003, 'DTCs' became 'TCs' in policy documents. We have not been able to find any discussion of the grounds for this change. It may have reflected no

more than a preference for a shorter title in 'branding' this initiative, but there may also have been other possible motives (see Chapter Four).

[3] Although many innovations adopting this type of approach to quality improvement in the NHS had already been underway, the government appeared to have embraced such approaches particularly warmly, notwithstanding some evidence that changes achieved might fall short of those hoped for (see, for example, Ham et al, 2003).

[4] By August 2004, patients waiting more than six months for elective surgery were intended to be offered a choice of provider, public or private, including TCs. Choice at referral was implemented for cataracts by January 2005, and generally at GP referral by December 2005 (Ricketts, 2003).

[5] There are suggestions in the healthcare construction literature that the pressure for rapid progress brought its own problems. For example, at an Architects for Health conference, a speaker from a firm involved with some London TCs was reported as saying that 'the politically driven programmes (from now until the next election)' caused difficulties because 'clients [had] little operational policy, no brief and no design, yet needing to open in 30 months.…This leads to a danger of building the wrong thing in haste. And construction has to start before design is finished, something we always used to try and avoid' (quoted in Architects for Health, 2003).

[6] In the healthcare construction literature, there are reports suggesting that the expected scale of the NHS-run TC programme under one financial programme was scaled back in 2003 in favour of full independent sector TC commissioning (see, for example, Anonymous, 2003).

[7] The Modernisation Agency was dissolved in 2005 and superseded by the NHS Institute for Innovation and Improvement, which has a similar remit to work with clinicians, NHS organisations, patients, the public, academia and industry to 'support the NHS to transform healthcare for patients and the public by rapidly developing and spreading new ways of working, new technology and world class leadership' and to promote a culture of innovation and lifelong learning.

TWO

Fertile ground? The organisational milieux of the treatment centres

'We recognise that what happens in the NHS ... is that every trust has resolved its own problem.' (Lakenfield senior manager)

Variation from beginning to end

Considering that this was supposed to be a unified national initiative, it was astonishing just how varied the eight case study sites turned out to be, not only in the manner in which the innovation occurred, but also in the configurations of the TCs themselves. Looking back, it should have been obvious that they would come in all shapes and sizes. After all, every previous central innovation of this kind, such as day surgery units in the 1980s or NHS Walk-in Centres in the 1990s, had spawned a mass of varied models. Indeed the Modernisation Agency had made clear that TCs *should* vary depending on local circumstances. But what they had in mind was the rational redesign of the same basic principles according to the likely demand for particular surgical services in localities with dissimilar populations. In fact the huge variety that emerged depended more on the happenstance of local organisational culture, politics, finances, relationships and buildings than on any rational analysis of local healthcare needs.

In order to understand this variety, and also to lay the foundations for understanding just what it was that shaped the innovation and its varied fate over time in different localities (see Table 2.1), we start by reviewing the initial conditions at each site. What kind of organisations were these NHS trusts that decided to become part of the early TC movement? How and why were they in a position to do so? We look here at each site in turn, examining both the internal circumstances and the external environment of each. Then, in the following chapter, where we examine their motives for opening a TC, we will be in a position to see not only how widely and why those reasons varied from place to place but also how wide-ranging they were in any particular hospital. Yet – as we shall see – despite this variety, there were also common features across the eight sites that will help us to understand how and why such an innovation evolves.

Table 2.1: A summary of the subsequent fates of the eight NHS TCs

	2006	2010
Ruckworth	Imminent closure due to insufficient patient numbers. Unless new tenants found, host trust faced with £5 million a year bill until lease expires	No longer an NHS TC. Premises rented out to private sector but still seen as major financial risk to host trust
Lakenfield	Phase I operating as a specialised ward, being used to maximise bed capacity and to spread new working methods in the host hospital. Phase II at planning stage, with arguments about the eventual size	New-build Phase II NHS TC very recently opened, linked physically to main hospital. Phase I beds transferred and absorbed into Phase II. Expecting 10,000 patients a year
Robbleswade	Beginning to operate after various teething problems as a TC that is being subsumed into large-scale hospital reconfiguration around planned care programmes	Operating as a 130-bed TC offering various surgical options and pre-assessment health checks prior to surgery integrated with main hospital
Stanwick	Struggling to find sufficient patients. Advertising for private companies to take over the management of the NHS TC and run it in the independent sector	National and local campaigns (and questionable financial viability) prevented, at the last minute, a sale to the private sector. Reconfigured NHS TC managed by local hospitals is now emerging as a leading centre for specialist elective surgery

Table 2.1: continued

	2006	2010
Brindlesham	Operating as stand-alone purpose-built NHS TC along lines of ACAD. Some links with independent sector integral in planning/ design	Still functioning as a stand-alone NHS TC, that also offers private sector operations alongside NHS care. Locally regarded as an excellent facility
St Urban's	Closed due to insufficient patient numbers	
Northendon	Struggling to find sufficient patients. Losing focus as a TC. Under severe financial pressure and further threatened by new nearby independent sector TC	Functioning as a well-appointed NHS TC with two operating theatres
Pollhaven	Reduced size and still struggling to find sufficient patients and to change working patterns	Operating as a small NHS TC (space for fewer than 30 patients) comprising a general medical and general surgical day case ward

Initial conditions

Ruckworth

When the call for TCs was issued, Ruckworth, an urban teaching hospital, was already in the midst of struggles to establish a stand-alone day surgery centre that was "separate … a little directorate on its own". Some years previously the hospital's entrepreneurial management team had already recognised that there might be a market to provide surgical services more widely, and when a local private hospital became available they had seized the opportunity to acquire it to house such a facility. It came as an unexpected bonus to find they could suddenly rebadge this somewhat risky venture as a flagship of the new national TC programme. Central funding and kudos would surely now follow. They quickly appointed a hospital manager from the private sector and a charismatic clinical director who shared the ambitions of breaking the NHS mould, importing a private sector mentality, and maximising their autonomy within the NHS. Using their considerable networks, this new team set about hand-picking clinical staff – many from private hospitals – as well as top local surgeons who would operate in the new unit. The new staff loved the place; small, friendly and beautifully appointed, it was, they said, "like a family". This close-knit unit was forging ahead and saw itself as a real 'trail blazer', overturning conventions to set up a whole new way of delivering services quite distinct from the rest of the hospital. The rhetoric was exactly in line with government policy (see Chapter One), including complete separation of elective patients, the radical streamlining of the service and full exploitation of the new Patient Choice scheme (see Chapter Four). But in their ambitious enthusiasm they did very little to keep the rest of the hospital, let alone other local NHS bodies, on board. Resentment at the TC's 'go-get-it' attitude was already growing among those who were outside the high-flying TC 'family'. Yet if it were to flourish the TC would need to rely heavily on the very people they were rapidly alienating.

It was not just the Ruckworth TC's cavalier attitude that was raising local antibodies. In a local health economy where most of the NHS was already struggling financially, the local primary care trusts (PCTs) found that a six-figure sum had been top sliced from their budgets to fund the new unit. Complex financial arrangements were set in place that neighbouring trusts were predicting (rightly as it turned out) would disadvantage the hospitals that were expected to send their patients to the new unit. Nearby hospitals felt that this new development meant not only that Ruckworth, as teaching hospitals do, was already taking their more complex and interesting patients, but now this new TC was also going to take their routine elective patients. What is more, it was cherry picking the top local surgeons. Some saw it, therefore, as a takeover bid destined to undermine other local hospitals in the whole area. It was hardly surprising, then, that when Ruckworth opened the doors of its beautifully refurbished ex-private hospital building to provide a single specialty TC for local NHS patients, there was little support from local trusts; indeed many were downright hostile.

Lakenfield

Lakenfield, a teaching hospital in a working-class area of a large city, could not have been more different from Ruckworth. The hospital had been under-performing for many years under lacklustre management, but a new chief executive was beginning to turn things around. Their main problems were first, an exceptionally long average stay for in-patients and second, an overstretched emergency service, which had major knock-on effects for their elective services. Their 'trolley wait' for patients admitted via casualty was unacceptably long, as was in-patient length of stay; moreover, a lack of space on the wards meant that elective operations were being cancelled at an intolerable rate. The new chief executive was determined to solve these problems by challenging organisational practices and myths that had long been part of the old regime; indeed his goal was to make Lakenfield a foundation hospital – a status only open to the best performing hospitals in the NHS. True to his reputation for being a hard man (which was contrary to his own view of being a "facilitative manager"), he soon replaced key senior staff and "sweated" them (his term) to work corporately and cohesively to produce new ideas. He reduced an inherited top tier of 30 managers to just three who directly reported to him, which led the rest of the organisation to feel distanced from the top team. There was a strong emphasis on a new set of core organisational values (with centrally written statements about openness, honesty, treating staff and patients with dignity and respect; striving for excellence, listening and encouraging feedback and so on) but some senior managers still worried about a lack of clear strategic direction. Some also felt pushed to solve their own problems with little concrete support.

Others, especially among the new team of clinical directors, saw this newly delegated power as a chance to challenge their senior clinical colleagues (mainly the consultant body) who were set in their ways. They fostered groups of imaginative and innovative doctors and nurses who were keen to improve things for patients and staff alike, some of whom were already using the bed crisis as an excuse to alter, very capably, the way treatment was delivered. This caucus of like-minded innovators were using their technical knowledge, enthusiasm and persuasiveness to gradually spread acceptance of new ways of practising. They were fostering ideas and values that included a 'can-do' mentality, a genuine desire to rethink practice, a determination to be patient-centred, an impatience with traditional professional boundaries and an openness to new ideas from other centres. Exploiting the concerns and enthusiasm of recalcitrant consultants so as to push them 'with the grain and not against it', they were unashamedly using their personal professional connections to reassure sceptical colleagues that they should trust in the changes. As a ginger group they had not only foreshadowed the government's modernisation agenda but had converted one of Lakenfield's wards to deal exclusively with elective and short-stay patients and were already seeing the benefits in falling 'trolley wait', length of stay and cancellation figures. As at Ruckworth, all of these approaches had predated the advent of the TC programme. But while Ruckworth was changing as a separate entity that stood outside the host hospital and was trying to leave it behind, the movers and shakers in Lakenfield were attempting from within to catalyse a change in the ethos of the entire hospital.

Externally these changes were invisible to the PCTs that sent their patients day to day to Lakenfield. Strategically, however, the hospital was embroiled in a major regional shake-up of services. It was the junior of two big university hospitals in a region that had been relatively poorly funded and lacking in strategic thinking. The region was now making amends with several large planning initiatives, most of which were based on strong aspirations to improve, and shift the emphasis towards, primary and community care. This attitude meant that there was little regional strategic thinking about developing hospital provision, which meant that all the hospitals were competitively carving out their own niches and their own futures.

Although the Lakenfield managers wanted to move ahead quickly to implement what was almost entirely an internal initiative – and moreover one that, thanks partly to personal contacts, had direct support from the Department of Health since it would not only help achieve targets but champion 'modernisation' – the region took several months to satisfy themselves that the bid was genuinely within the spirit of the TC programme. They eventually accepted Phase I of the TC project, which was just an enhanced version of the existing successful elective and short-stay ward. However, the Phase II plans to open a fully fledged TC three years later along the lines of the ACAD became ensnarled in a growing tussle between the push towards rationalising services across the region and the need for the hospital to solve its own performance problems and establish the space for it to keep its role as a leading teaching hospital in the city. Indeed, it was to be some 10 years after Phase I was officially opened as part of the TC programme that the Phase II new-build took over as the hospital's TC (see Table 2.1).

Robbleswade

Robbleswade, housed in a brand new hospital in a market town, contrasted strongly with the hard-driven management cultures of Ruckworth and Lakenfield. Recovering from the upheaval of the recent move to the new building, the Robbleswade managers who would be responsible for designing the TC betrayed a tangible sense of 'planning fatigue'. Their weariness with changes to the hospital that had not lived up to their promise undermined from the very start the way they set about planning their TC. The chief executive who had overseen the move to the new hospital had recently accepted the fresh challenge of running a rival hospital and had taken some key top managers with him. Others also soon left, leaving rumblings about careerists who had used the opening of new hospital as a stepping stone and had not stayed to see the move through. As their replacements were still finding their feet, many staff members felt there was no clear management strategy other than fire fighting, and that they were lurching from one crisis to the next. There were vacancies in several key operational roles coupled with a lack of clarity about who should be driving service change. The result was a tendency for consensus decisions that – because they were in fact rarely backed by the whole team – often led to paralysed inaction.

Nevertheless as a new hospital they felt that despite the problems of managing all their other priorities their hospital would lose face – and competitive edge – if they did not apply for a TC. Unlike Ruckworth, the TC's internal structures were closely, often inseparably, linked with those of the host hospital. For example, bed planning discussions about the TC were integral to discussions about bed configuration across the whole hospital. At all the meetings about the TC the key managers also held posts in the trust or the hospital, which led to what they liked to call a "whole system approach". It also meant, however, that the TC planning process was denied the focus and attention it needed until (at the strategic health authority's [SHA's] suggestion) a project manager was appointed, which gave the TC project more consistency and drive. Also unlike Ruckworth, relations with the SHA were good; it played an important role, as the intervention over the project manager suggests, in helping to shape the planning of the TC. Initially, the local PCT, which was also fully on board with the idea of the new unit, was expected to provide 95 per cent of the TC's patients. However, two other neighbouring PCTs, whence came most of the other five per cent, were unhappy with the performance of their usual hospital and so agreed to begin sending all their elective patients to Robbleswade. This agreement, which was expected in the future to supply around half of the expected TC's patients, formed a key part of the original TC plans but later, as we shall see, turned out to be a treacherous miscalculation.

Initially, however, the main problems lay elsewhere. Having just built a hospital, Robbleswade had good relations with the private finance initiative (PFI) contractor and the builders. So the process of constructing the new TC was in essence a re-run of the hospital building project on a smaller scale. The downside was that the hospital was therefore the focus of a great deal of hostility from the NHS trade unions, who objected to the whole principle of PFI and subjected Robbleswade to a sustained local campaign against privatisation. Nevertheless the new build went ahead.

Stanwick

Long before the government's new TC programme, several local trusts that suffered very poor services in a particular surgical specialty had agreed to join forces in sponsoring Stanwick as a small, stand-alone centre to provide top notch care for that single specialty. Stanwick's management team had close links with a surgicenter in the US (see Chapter One), whose mentorship was strongly influencing their philosophy. From the start the Stanwick team used organisational development groups and imported managers to create a new culture of a 'high performing organisation with high performing people'. Three other key aspirational values were declared: '(1) caring for patients, families and staff, a learning organisation, (2) embracing continuous improvement, and pursuing excellence, (3) measures and outcomes' (Stanwick internal document). Stanwick invited dozens of hospital consultants from five hospitals to work at the centre, where they might be asked to operate on patients other than their own – acting in essence as skilled surgical technicians. But a major feature at Stanwick was the intention that the broader aspects of patient care would be led by nurses with new skills to take on many of the clinical roles traditionally performed by doctors and other professions.

Stanwick therefore, like Ruckworth, was a single specialty centre, driven by a strong and ambitious management team that wanted the TC to have a separate independent existence imbued with the values of the private sector. However, whereas Ruckworth was several miles from its parent organisation, Stanwick was housed in a wing of the parent hospital on which it relied heavily for support services. Many of Stanwick's top team were unhappy with that arrangement: they wanted to throw off the yoke of their parent hospital. The result was a tense compromise described officially as "recognising a degree of quasi-autonomous operational independence", which in practice led to continuous quarrels about Stanwick's freedom to bend NHS personnel and other rules. Such freedom was crucial because the top team, who revelled in the rhetoric of "throwing away the rule book", demanded to "employ our own [and] start as we mean to go on", not least because they intended to recruit and train a new cadre of nurse practitioner. But more generally, like Ruckworth, they wanted ruthlessly to break what they saw as the stagnant mould of NHS culture (and consultant power). In fact their attitude was very much in line with central government's modernisation agenda of nurse-led patient pathways and related initiatives. Yet rather than being allowed to take it forward they felt that they were being held back by the parent hospital, who seemed always to be frowning on their innovative ideas, demanding justification, and delaying progress. For example, when the Stanwick TC tried to recruit to new nursing roles that did not fit in with existing staff gradings, the parent hospital's managers "went ballistic" and the TC had to fall back into line.

There were some parallels with Ruckworth; TC managers at Stanwick felt that the host hospital was not merely questioning innovative practices but was positively cynical about the venture, unduly apprehensive of the risks, resentful that the TC was poaching some of the best staff, envious that it was receiving special favours and secretly hoping it would fail. Some of the local PCTs' chief executives who had originally signed up to the Stanwick scheme had long gone and been replaced by new managers who, frustratingly for Stanwick, needed to have the underlying concepts sold to them all over again. For their part the hospital and local PCTs maintained that Stanwick was failing to deal with genuine concerns over clinical governance and risk management for a nurse-led service whose very idea had raised many an eyebrow among local clinicians. They felt they needed the "rule book" to restrain a gung ho, semi-autonomous, nurse-led unit that they worried might otherwise go awry. And even if it did not, they fretted that, for example, post-operative patients might be sent home too early, putting undue pressure on community services. Stanwick tried to be "meticulous" in dealing with these concerns but for all sorts of reasons communications were unsatisfactory and – despite the support of the regional authority and the local workforce confederation responsible for nurse training – key external stakeholders believed that deeply held concerns remained unresolved.

In some respects, therefore, the resulting tensions resembled Ruckworth's, but there were also some parallels with Robbleswade. The TC had ambitions to bring in patients from beyond the neighbouring PCTs and hospitals by becoming a major supplier of services across the entire city and beyond; initial negotiations under the Patient Choice scheme suggested that this would be a fertile source of patients. However, this was never to materialise.

Brindlesham

Brindlesham had two acute hospitals that were part of an extensive trust encompassing a market town. To try and deal with an overspend and long waiting lists, the trust had rationalised its services by closing the acute and emergency services in one of the hospitals and leaving it just as an "elective hospital". Local dismay and anger thrust Brindlesham into a political glare that would not go away. Moreover, staff felt that the trust was disjointed, with little cohesion between the two hospitals. Frequent changes of personnel at senior trust management level, including more than one change of chief executive, exacerbated the fragmentary feel of an organisation with no clear or consistent direction. Yet despite the lack of focus, the organisation was not risk averse; indeed there were many resourceful innovators at both sites who were keen to try and put things right, if only out of a sense of loyalty to their own hospital if not to the trust as a whole.

No sooner had the idea of a TC been conceived than a project manager with experience of ambulatory care (see Chapter One) was appointed. He took advantage of the slack links between the trust's constituent parts to construct an organisation within an organisation, "a semi-autonomous business unit", which – unlike Stanwick's "quasi-autonomous operational independence" – succeeded. Under his clear leadership the TC increased its independence and offered a space where new ideas could be tested and encouraged to flourish. It helped, of course, that many saw the investment in an exciting new TC at the "elective hospital" as an elegant way of appeasing the local community who wanted their hospital back. However, the project manager's vision for the TC was also an important motivating factor. Through his extensive previous experience and knowledge of ambulatory care and his close networks with the world of TCs he brought both authority and credibility. When he echoed the slogans of the TC movement by saying that TCs are about "transforming patients" experiences' by focusing on "a wellness model", in which the patient "isn't ill but just needs fixing", most of the Brindlesham team supported him. In short, and in contrast to many of the other case study sites, Brindlesham had visionary and credible transformational leadership and was quickly functioning as an integrated but relatively independent and thoroughly different organisation within an organisation. Despite some initial teething problems with timing and design, Brindlesham staff were determined from the start to make it a showcase TC.

Unlike Stanwick or Ruckworth, the project leader was careful in the midst of the turbulent local politics to foster harmonious relations with the SHA and local PCTs, which soon signed up to having a TC on the site of the 'elective hospital'; it might not only placate the local activists but also, they hoped, help tackle all those challenging government targets such as waiting list reductions. Indeed so enthusiastic was their involvement on the board of the TC that the Brindlesham PCT tried (ultimately unsuccessfully) to take it over. In resisting this attempt to confine the TC to the immediate vicinity, the Brindlesham TC, with strong support from the health authority, spread its net much more widely to capitalise on the renewed NHS emphasis on consumer choice and to encourage distant trusts to send their patients. Those far-flung PCTs had mixed feelings: yes the TC might help them get their patients treated more quickly but on the other hand, the costs of sending them to Brindlesham seemed inordinately high, even compared to local private providers. So although they initially contracted to send their patients, some did not renew those commitments the following year.

St Urban's

A large teaching hospital within a major city, St Urban's was renowned for its 'can do', action-driven culture of opportunism, innovation and risk taking. Always trying to be ahead of the game, St Urban's was, for example, at the forefront of electronic patient records, of the new wave of acquisition of private hospital premises and later of foundation hospitals. But many of its middle managers complained that in falling over itself to be out front, the hospital often acted on intuition and assumptions rather than analysis and facts. They saw the senior managers as being too easily attracted to the "policy flavour of the month", leaving other people to pick up the pieces as their own attention "moved on to the next Big Idea". Within the hospital, many used the word "tribal" to describe not only the segmented and autonomous clinical groups that were happy to let each other sink or swim as long as their own fiefdom was thriving, but also the relations between managers and clinicians. Even though some senior doctors were themselves highly effective, innovative, charismatic managers, many doctors and managers held traditional NHS attitudes of mutual antagonism. Doctors might typically characterise managers (who in their view were often transient, inexperienced and naïve) as failing to consult and communicate, while the managers would often stereotype the consultant body as egotistical, recalcitrant and a powerful obstruction to change.

Like Ruckworth, St Urban's had an adversarial, some said paranoid, culture about a local health economy that they saw as sending them "rubbish patients", withholding information, trying to deflect resources from them, or otherwise slowing them down in their drive to innovate. This pervasive 'them and us' attitude, with its derogatory stereotypes of local stakeholders and its caricatures of a mediocre and stick-in-the-mud 'centre' of the NHS, had led to longstanding tensions. The hospital preferred to steer its own path, paying as little attention as possible to the rest of the health economy. As a result, neighbouring organisations saw St Urban's as arrogant and predatory in its relentless quest for glory. However, because patients came to the hospital from a very wide range of sources, the hospital was less reliant on any particular local PCT than, say, Lakenfield or Robbleswade, and therefore felt less vulnerable to PCT pressure.

At the many meetings between St Urban's and key local potential stakeholders the TC was rarely mentioned. Maybe this was because there was so much else to discuss, but maybe also, as some suggested, St Urban's adversarial and competitive attitude may have led its managers to keep their cards close to their chest. Whatever the reason, its neighbours and feeder PCTs later felt deliberately excluded from any decision making about the planned TC. PCTs still played very little role in commissioning care at that stage and St Urban's negotiations about the TC, such as they were, were mainly confined to the SHA and the Department of Health. Indeed when the local PCT did later get more involved, St Urban's simultaneously, and without the trust's knowledge, negotiated via the Patient Choice scheme to get additional patients at a different rate of payment, leading to a flurry of accusations and counter-accusations of spurious billing and 'double counting' of patients, which was symptomatic of the lack of trust between the commissioners and the hospital. In short, St Urban's, a visibly successful hospital, was seen both internally and in its external relations as ambitious, risk-taking, competitive, uncooperative, seat-of the-pants, individualist and riven with tensions.

Northendon

Northendon was located on the outskirts of a small holiday resort now long past its heyday. It was a relatively small hospital that in many ways, mirroring the faded grandeur of the resort, was a backwater that needed to pull itself into the mainstream if it was to thrive. A traditional doctor-led hierarchy played a powerful role, and even consultant surgeons – who are not generally known for their love of "NHS bureaucracy" – were heard to say that the place was under-managed. The relatively small management staff, also very hierarchical, sent most decisions upwards to the director of finance and chief executive, the two of whom had a working partnership that went a long way back. There was a clear sense from the staff that personal contact with this duumvirate was a key to getting things done. The smallness of the hospital made this possible; there was a lot of "popping into the office" to talk to the chief executive. Northendon Hospital was seen from outside as rather traditional – even backward – with too few managers trying to cover too much ground and using time-honoured paper-based administrative methods, which meant that they were usually slower than other hospitals in meeting the demands of the higher levels of the NHS. Dealings were nevertheless generally very harmonious with the local PCTs, who were all satisfied that they had input into the planning of the TC. The SHA was supportive too; indeed they were its catalyst. When Northendon's managers originally mooted opening a day surgical unit, it was the health authority that suggested doubling its capacity by applying instead for funding from the national TC programme, despite their concerns – which had to be taken account of – that the new facility might weaken the position of a nearby teaching hospital.

The initial thinking about the TC was led by a small team of middle managers variously seconded to this task. They mainly did this work as overtime on top of their other duties. This small part-time team had – and created around them – a real sense of common purpose, team working, and many features of an action learning set or community of practice. They were zealously committed to the project and later often glowingly recalled the final hectic run-up opening the unit on time. One of the foundation myths of the TC, highly evocative of the organisational culture, was of the chair of the hospital board coming in personally to hang pictures on the walls the day before the grand opening when a cleaner, not recognising him with a hammer in his hand, shouted at him for creating dust. Thus within the very traditional history and homely structure of the trust, there were people keen to get behind the change and push it forwards. However, they later each returned to the jobs they had been doing before their involvement in setting up the TC and the skills they brought to the project were not developed nor built upon, reinforcing the view that this was not an organisation ready to recognise, reward and develop good staff. Northendon, in short, was a small town hospital with an old-fashioned NHS administrative culture, under-managed, subject to the medical hierarcey, and reliant for change on a group of enthusiasts.

Pollhaven

Two hospitals with very different cultures had recently merged at Pollhaven, which, like Northendon, was a holiday resort past its hey-day. As at Brindlesham, the reconfiguration of health services meant that one of the hospitals – the one at Pollford, the smaller hospital where the TC would eventually be based – was designated for elective activity only. Pollford had a reputation as a hospital with top-down managers and acquiescent staff, which deterred those who were being asked to move from the larger Havenshore Hospital to Pollford. For their part, the staff at Pollford perceived the reconfiguration as part of the larger Havenhsore's inevitable "takeover" of their hospital. Inevitably, these early tensions were to have a direct effect on the development of the TC.

When Pollhaven's managers proposed that the elective services should be recast as a TC, the doctors, who were a strong force in both sites, resisted. They dug their heels in about the 20-minute drive between the sites, about the prospect of working in unfamiliar environments, about having to cede control over the booking system for their operating lists, and so on.

Nursing staff and managers were better disposed than the doctors to the merger and to the idea of using Pollford Hospital just for elective surgery, but neither they nor the more senior managers felt empowered or found it easy to push for the change. Post-merger Pollhaven's chief problem was defiance by a consultant body that the managers generally felt unable to persuade. There was also a sense that while some individuals were positive about the TC there was a general lack of ownership by staff. Worse, not one senior consultant was prepared to champion the idea of a separate site for cold (elective) surgery. Nevertheless the TC plans went ahead

The trust then tried to steer clear of trouble by proposing that instead of having separate "hot" (acute) and "cold" hospitals, there should be a TC on both sites, but external bodies such as the region and local PCTs disagreed. Indeed the plans for the TC were constrained very early on, before an outline business case was even begun, by a strategic overview of services being carried out at the regional level. So a single TC it had to be, after which the region and the commissioners regarded the setting up of the TC as largely an internal matter. They played little further part, even though the two main PCTs each contributed a five-figure sum to improve staffing for the new unit. The plan was to fly in teams of surgeons from overseas to carry out the operations in the TC, but the commissioning PCTs allowed funding, staffing and clinical governance to be integral with the overall internal strategy that Pollhaven was setting for itself. This also meant, however, that when the Pollhaven TC was later to run into financial difficulties, it was subject to management reorganisations and financial retrenchment over which the host trust had sole control. The financial setbacks resulted in a significant scaling down of the planned operation of the TC and frustration among those responsible within it for delivering the intended improvements and modernisation of service.

Given the rhetoric that the government was pushing across the NHS about strategic planning and about the pivotal role of PCTs in shaping health care provision, such a lack of serious engagement between the PCTs and hospitals over the planning of TCs was surprising. Yet not just at Pollhaven, but also others such as Lakenfield, external stakeholders played little part in planning these local initiatives; indeed in others such as Ruckworth and St Urban's there was outright hostility from the planning stage onwards. During this initial phase of development such distant or antagonistic relations with local PCTs and neighbouring trusts had little real effect on the emergent TCs, who simply got on with the task of opening their doors to patients. But as we shall show, the external relations took on greater significance as the TCs got under way.

Initial conditions: taking stock

Having surveyed the initial conditions at each of the sites, what have we learnt? In terms of their internal environments, each trust had its distinctive managerial style, aspirations, problems and relationships. Organisationally, there was little that the host trusts had in common. All had key staff with what several interviewees called a "can-do mentality" who included – for whatever varying motives – some who were willing and able champions of the innovation. But then, so do most large organisations. Perhaps the only other feature they all shared was that a TC appeared to be both necessary and timely to help solve some organisational problem or achieve some local aim or other – and not just the aim of improving the care of elective patient.

In terms of their external environments, again we have found little in common. Relationships with external stakeholder ranged from the adversarial and hostile dealings at Ruckworth and St Urban's, through to the harmonious and constructive partnerships at Brindlesham or Northendon. In between these extremes was apparent disinterest (Lakenfield) or a mixture of tense and supportive relationships (for instance, with the local hospital partners at Stanwick, or with PCTs at Robbleswade). Within that wide variety of external environments, however, the one thing that all the sites had was a deep-rooted set of (different) *local* historical and cultural roots that were to pay a crucial role in the early stages of establishing a TC.

THREE

Taking up the challenge: local motives for the innovation

'If you were to have this conversation with any of the "management" guys, they'll tell you the right gobbledygook, and tell you that we're absolutely committed to that [modernisation]. In reality, we're so struggling to get the work and get through it and stay afloat financially, that that's not the agenda as I perceive it.' (senior clinical manager, St Urban's)

Chapter Two highlighted the paradox that, considering all eight sites were part of the same NHS and engaging with the same national innovation programme, their initial circumstances had almost nothing in common with each other. However, they all had local justifications for opening a TC that were the result of complex 'negotiations' between different 'players' at each site, each of whom interpreted the innovation differently. At each site, key players in the early phases of the development of the TCs contested their understandings and definitions of a TC and what it might mean for the organisation. The tussles, disagreements and bargaining that would shape the resulting TCs were not simple interprofessional (often referred to as "tribal") battles between, say, doctors, managers and nurses. Rather than splitting along professional lines, they seemed rather to fall into four types of player, namely opportunists, pragmatists, idealists and sceptics, who were to be found in varying proportions in each of the sites. Each type had a role in determining the fate of the innovation, using different aspects of the local initial conditions in each site to argue the case for or against developing a TC (Pope et al, 2006).[1]

Opportunists, pragmatists, idealists and sceptics

Opportunists saw TCs as a chance to do something (rebuild, expand, renew) that they might not otherwise have the chance to do, which was often an innovation they had already been planning or developing. In several of our sites opportunists used the TC programme as a way to get capital funding to finance projects they had long been hoping to implement. At Northendon, for example, a project group had, for a long time, been wanting to expand day surgery in their hospital. Following the announcement of TC funding and prodded by the SHA, the project group developed a bid for a TC mainly as a vehicle for the day surgery unit they had thus far been unable to realise. Lakenfield was another example where opportunists seized the day, recognising that the TC programme was a chance not only to provide a new facility that would relieve the overstretched hospital's crippling bed shortages but also to refurbish a costly 1970s building, long regarded as a millstone that was under-used because it was tied up as outdated, outsourced hospital accommodation. Housing a new TC in that building would resolve these twin problems of an overstretched in-patient service and an under-used building. At Ruckworth, the opportunists had already grabbed the chance to buy up a private hospital when it had come up for sale, but were struggling to establish it as a single specialty surgical unit. When the TC programme was then fortuitously announced, it was obvious that this was the opportunity to provide the impetus – and cash injection – to make that idea a reality. And at Stanwick, opportunists who had been planning a separate nurse-led specialist surgical facility likewise saw their chance to link it to the TC programme and thereby gain both money and political support.

Pragmatists focused on local, practical matters, notably delivering appropriate care and meeting the required performance targets. They were gradual reformers, not radical revolutionaries. The pragmatic perspective was about the business of simply getting on with delivering a good service. While care might well be improved in line with the modernisation ideal enshrined in government policy, the main intention for the pragmatists was not to rethink practice but simply to streamline or otherwise upgrade it. They recognised that a TC afforded an opportunity to do so and perhaps also have the bonus of being in the spotlight of a major initiative that would make that work more visible and more rewarding. But the pragmatism of simply using the TC as a chance to bring about long-desired improvements under a new banner could easily spill over into a more idealist frame of mind. In Lakenfield, for example, there were many pragmatists who did little more than use the innovation as a way to further develop services they were already providing. But that TC also allowed a group of innovative idealists to ride the wave of modernisation and push others, including the pragmatists, towards radically new ways of working.

Idealists fervently embraced the broader vision and underlying philosophy of TCs such as the 'modernisation agenda' of professional reform and (although they might eschew the term) 're-engineered patient pathways'. In many sites the idealists were the powerhouse for developing radical new ways of working and for persuading colleagues to adopt them. They used their position and authority if they were senior staff, or just their guile and organisational skills if they were more junior, to promulgate a different way of thinking among their colleagues. The idealists at Lakenfield, for example, achieved this partly by running a training course on process mapping, which got staff collectively and systematically to rethink from first principles the processes to which patients were subjected. The course, once it was opened up to wide range of hospital staff, became a vehicle through which two relatively junior but inspirational managers led the spread of the ideas that enabled the TC to redesign the delivery of care and engender an important shift in mentality across the whole hospital. At Brindlesham, in contrast, the chief idealist was the very senior project manager who was known to be fully wedded to the ideology of modernisation and "transforming patients" experiences', which indeed was why he had been hired specifically to shape the establishment of an innovative TC.

Sceptics also played a big role, not least by tempering the zeal of the idealists and opportunists and urging caution. (Of course in some sites that we did not study because no TC was opened, they doubtless won the argument – as they had nearly done in some of our sample.) More risk-averse or possibly just more jaded about yet more change in the NHS, it was the sceptics who viewed TCs as transient fads or, worse, as dangerous risks, and who therefore resisted the change. Adopting such a viewpoint, sceptics could be powerful players in shaping the development of individual TCs. At Robbleswade such scepticism was linked to the "planning fatigue" brought about by the recent opening of the new hospital. Often, though, the scepticism was more deep rooted and generic. Sceptics often suspected that the rationale for TCs went beyond – or even had little to do with – the philosophy of TCs as portrayed by the government or championed by the idealists. They saw it instead as simply another unwanted organisational change imposed by 'the centre' or as part of broader (party) political manoeuvring. Others were simply more cautious; for example the concerns at Stanwick were largely about the possible unintended impact of nurse-led care on risk management in the TC.

We now turn to examine the reasons why, at all our case study sites, the sceptics lost the initial argument and a TC was opened. The potential for opening a TC had many attractions. Naturally, the key motivating factors in each site were steeped in the initial circumstances (Chapter Two), which moulded the arguments about the local pros and cons that were thrashed out as the plans for each TC took shape. The incentives can be divided into three groups, which we call 'Improving quality', such as better patient experience or professional practices, 'Improving quantity', such as cuts in waiting lists or raised cost-efficiency and/or income, and 'Improving kudos', such as enhanced reputation, profile and influence, both organisational and personal. These motivating forces could often co-exist within a single site, sometimes pulling in the same direction and sometimes not, since inevitably key actors and factions held differing, sometimes inconsistent arguments for and against their TC.

The interplay between the motivation to improve quality, quantity and kudos was therefore not always straightforward. At Pollhaven for example, it was clear that something had to change if the hospital was to meet its performance targets, and many believed that a TC was just what was needed to improve the efficiency and the quality of care. Yet some clinicians were arguing that it was clinically inappropriate to use one of the hospitals entirely for elective care, an argument that managers interpreted as masking the consultants' wish to cling to well-established working conditions and practices. At St Urban's, apart from a small group of modernisation enthusiasts, there was little emphasis on the TC's role in improving the quality of patient care by modernising care pathways, and still less on the prospect of reforming professional roles and attitudes. What really mattered – and so much so that it made the TC an imperative – was the fact that a TC would improve the financial and political standing of the hospital. At Lakenfield, on the other hand, a number of influential players were keen to use the TC to break the mould of traditional professional practice and modernise care (improving quality), and moreover there was almost unanimous agreement that a TC would be a pragmatic way to help rectify failing performance levels such as waiting times (improving quantity). But although the Lakenfield TC *per se* might be all but invisible to the local health economy, the kudos arising from its impact on quantity and quality would give the hospital essential political leverage in maintaining its position in the planned redistribution of hospital services across the region. So the various motives underlying the emergence and development of each TC, whether acting in concert or in opposition to each other, differed not only between the sites but also within them.

The key lesson as we explore the examples is that even a centrally led initiative like the TC programme will inevitably become embroiled in, and grow out of, the local concerns and struggles. While the government and Department of Health may have had their view of what TCs should be like, what emerged was chiefly a series of local solutions to local problems.

Improving quality

Patient care

One of the main motivators, even for many of the sceptics, was the chance that a TC would be a way to improve patient experience. Some, especially the idealists and pragmatists, were fired up by the reports of good practice that were buzzing around the clinical and managerial networks of the NHS and by the broader drive towards modernisation of care processes urged by *The NHS Plan* (see Chapter One, this volume). These developments all conspired to give key players in each of our sites the incentive to use the TC as a means to improve care in innovative and radical ways. Often this was described, especially by enthusiasts, as the "new ways of working"; exciting ideas that ranged from standardised, evidence-based, patient-centred care, through integrated care pathways, through one-stop multi-professional clinics, to simply having a way to prevent emergency admissions from overwhelming elective services.

Stanwick, for example, anticipated benefits in patient care that included greater predictability of the processes that they would undergo, which would allow greater levels of preparation and smoother transfers, and the development of services closer to home, especially post-acute rehabilitation. With an eye to the new cadre of nurse practitioner, Stanwick also expected to achieve clinical benefits such as enhanced training opportunities and increasing specialist expertise among nurses, better quality control and the more efficient use of consultant surgeons and anaesthetists, all of which were expected to result in better care. There were many similar examples among the other sites, but sometimes the simple desire to improve care was tempered by other motives. At St Urban's, for example, the idealist senior staff who did talk about their intention to modernise services and review the skill mix were aware that *being seen* to put the patient first was a key to surviving in an increasingly competitive local health economy in which other hospitals, and even more so the private sector, were improving the patient experience in order to attract referrals. Any idealism at St Urban's was, in other words, detectably laced with more pragmatic self-interest.

Reforming professional practices

The new ways of working had a number of spin-offs that some key players saw as being more important than the new unit itself. Foremost among these was the longstanding desire to reform the way clinicians did their jobs – not only in terms of their day-to-day management of patient care but also in the way they related to other professions and to the hospital as a whole. For many in the health service this seemed an opportunity to break down barriers, alter the range and combination of skills of a whole new generation of nurses and allied clinical professions and increase their autonomy and power. If nothing else, it was a potential way of bringing some recalcitrant hospital consultants to heel.

The TC was often seen as a route to reforming, by example and knock-on effect, the way the whole hospital delivered services. At Lakenfield staff from the TC were not only running the process-mapping course that was gradually transforming care throughout the hospital, but also demonstrating to sceptical surgeons how much better their operating schedules and waiting lists could be organised, and how much the new approach to care was improving their patients' experience. In contrast, would-be stand-alone TCs such as Ruckworth, Stanwick or Brindlesham had given up on the idea of introducing the new ways of working in what the TC visionaries saw as their irredeemably hidebound host hospitals. They saw their strength in trying to maintain as much separation as possible. At Stanwick, for example, the feeling, especially among the converts who had been to the US surgicenter, was that the necessary changes could only be made by starting with a clean sheet away from the main hospital and free of the ties of established custom and practice. But the aim was still the same – to radically alter professional roles and practice.

TCs also provided the opportunity to modernise the professional roles of clinicians other than doctors. In particular, many TCs hoped to broaden the skills of nurses, operating theatre staff, professions allied to medicine (such as physiotherapists) and occasionally also radiographers. Northendon idealists were keen, for example, to find new ways of using assistant practitioners and moving nurses between the TC and other areas to increase their skills and range of competencies. Their Robbleswade counterparts spoke of introducing pre-assessment clinics and using surgical assistants in the operating theatre. Others were getting non-doctors to be able to order X-rays, prescribe, discharge patients, and generally be able to take on each other's roles to suit the patients' (and hospital's) needs rather than sticking to traditional professional boundaries. Moreover they were very keen to allow non-medical staff to take full control of booking patients for operations. Just how these new roles and arrangements eventually developed – or not – will be dealt with more fully in Chapter Six.

In the early days, and often linked to the ideal of changing established clinical roles and behaviours, there were some idealists who saw their TC as a chance to inculcate new ways of working and new attitudes into young clinicians training there. For the pragmatists too, TCs were a place where more efficient training might take place, since trainee clinicians would see lots of the same sorts of patient, and so become very slick at routine surgical techniques and their associated care pathways. Maybe also, argued some, TCs could be unique research opportunities; given that they treated so many similar routine patients, controlled trials would be easier. But the sceptics, whose voices became louder as some TCs developed, worried that routine 'factory' processing of patients would damage medical training and staff development by stripping all the routine patients out of the teaching hospitals where such training was concentrated. (This argument was later also to be levelled by professional organisations as part of their national campaigns against the independent sector TCs.)

Optimising local premises

TCs could also provide a chance to deal with concerns about facilities. The concerns fell into three main categories: optimising bed use; a chance to upgrade existing premises; and a way of paying for a new building that the hospital already knew (or thought it knew) it needed. Northendon had all three; the trust saw the opportunity not only to improve its bed management, upgrade their building and establish a separate unit but also in one fell swoop to increase income by batching groups of patients and types of operation together in a state-of-the-art day case unit. The new facility would not only treat Northendon patients more efficiently, but act as a magnet for surgical cases on waiting lists in distant localities, thereby increasing its income and viability. Long before the TC programme there were stop-start discussions as various designs were talked about, including a stand-alone facility. Some of the early key players went out on fact finding trips to see how other hospitals did day care. They came back brimming with ideas and became agitators for a day care unit. A windfall legacy from a local philanthropist enabled the opportunist chairman, whose general philosophy was 'let's just get on and do it', to push though the building of a two-storey "shell", even though it was still unclear how the money would be found to fit it out as a day care unit. This later proved decisive; having that empty space was suddenly a boon when the call came for bids to open TCs. The final piece fell into place from higher up the NHS hierarchy, not least politicians, who desperately needed some early wins for the TC programme and the waiting list initiative. When they learned that there was already an empty new shell that could rapidly be converted into a state-of-the art TC to deal with the local waiting lists and provide a shining example of NHS success, they smoothed the release of funds to open the TC on condition that the unit was up and running within a very short time. This serendipitous melding of central and local motives meant that once Northendon had struck the deal, they faced a precipitous and nerve-wracking deadline that was met with a derring-do spirit by the whole team – as in the story of Northendon's hammer-wielding, dust-raising chairman (see Chapter Two).

There were many other examples of the TC being a solution to local lack of suitable space. Lakenfield, for example, was able to solve its pressing need to recommission a white elephant of a 1970s building. Pollhaven already knew that it needed new premises; the case for the TC to upgrade poor quality premises was obvious to all. But the fraught local politics called for great care to avoid the pitfalls that came from the factional vying between the two hospitals that were being merged. Northendon had been looking for a way to solve the clinicians' complaints that in-patients, surgical day cases and medical outliers were all crowded together on their wards, making it difficult to protect day case space and enable day surgery to be done efficiently. The case was therefore already made not only for a clearly defined space in which to siphon the routine in-patient load away from the main hospital, ring-fencing day surgery, but also to provide much-needed potential space for any future increases in numbers.

Improving staffing

Another benefit of opening a TC, often mentioned by pragmatists, was its potential to attract good staff, not just because the added work called for more staff but because the new ways of working would attract more go-ahead people to those posts. St Urban's, for example, were able to employ several new consultant anaesthetists and surgeons on the strength of opening a TC (even though, as we shall see, the unit ultimately attracted far fewer patients than they had expected.) At Robbleswade and Lakenfield, where there was a history of difficulties in recruiting particular types of staff such as theatre technicians and nurses, the development of the TC was seen as feeding into a larger process of role redesign, which could systematically address skill (and staff) shortages. Role redesign was promoted as a way of changing professional practice and the whole culture of the hospital. At Stanwick, the strong emergent identity of the centre as a nurse-led unit, incorporating advanced training and good prospects for career progression for nursing staff, was used to sell the TC to prospective staff during the initial recruitment phase and subsequent education of a cohort of advanced nurse practitioners with newly enhanced status.

Improving quantity

Meeting performance targets

Senior managers in all eight trusts were strongly driven to open a TC because they saw it as a way to meet the NHS performance targets that were becoming both increasingly prominent and progressively more challenging. The need to reduce waiting times and waiting lists was everywhere a key incentive to open a TC – and in this regard the local views about the role of a TC coincided well with those of the government (see Chapter One). Often the trusts saw the potential for the new TC to reduce waiting lists as being principally about increasing capacity so as to increase throughput.

But the TC could also help meet other targets. At Lakenfield, for example, the really urgent performance problem was to reduce the unacceptable wait that patients were having after admission via the accident and emergency (A&E) department. This had become a critical problem for the hospital, a consequence of insufficient beds on the wards for emergencies to be admitted. The shortage of in-patient beds was partly due to inefficient planning of admissions and discharges of elective patients, who in turn were being shuffled around the wards to try and make space for emergency patients. Moreover, elective patients would all too often be cancelled because there was no bed for them. The opening of a TC was the missing element that allowed the hospital not only to manage the elective patients more efficiently, but also to provide short-term space in which to move patients when they did not need emergency care – hardly the intended role of a TC, but an unmissable opportunity nonetheless for Lakenfield.

Improving provision of services across the locality

Several of the sites were attracted by the prospect of taking on some of the elective work of neighbouring trusts that were known to be having difficulties meeting their waiting list targets. This also made TCs attractive to many PCTs as a way to increase local capacity across the whole of the local health economy and so improve access to services. Many saw this as the key to meeting targets set by *The NHS Plan*. At Robbleswade, for example, the shortfall of the new hospital's capacity had to be rectified as soon as possible or several of the surrounding PCT managers' necks would be on the line. At Northendon too there were significant gaps in the local provision that needed urgently plugging. Having failed to find anywhere even quite distant that could offer the surgical services they needed, the PCT was at the point of considering purchasing a mobile theatre and staffing it with locum surgeons. So when the Northendon trust suggested opening a TC the PCTs were only too glad to support the proposal.

At Stanwick, all the local organisations (hospitals and PCTs) shared the same problem in one key surgical sub-specialty: there were not enough beds, theatre lists or surgeons to do all the work required. Indeed the possibility of a shared centre that would deal with all the elective patients from all the participating trusts had been fruitlessly under discussion since the mid-1990s. The chance to open a TC at Stanwick was an ideal way to realise this long-held aspiration and thereby release capacity for over 3,000 operations in other surgical specialties at the participating trusts. It would reduce waiting time, help meet targets, improve access and give better value for money by centralising the service. What was not stated in the public pronouncements was that the TC would also be a good way for Stanwick to divert funding from the neighbouring trusts to open a unit that was already part of their strategic plan.

The proposal for separating elective and emergency care at Pollhaven had also originally come out of a series of major reviews of services and capital investments begun some five years earlier across the two constituent trusts it now comprised. However, the newly merged trust was fearful of the public and staff reaction that would explode if they restricted emergency care to just one of the hospitals, leaving the other free for elective care. Nevertheless the various reviews had pushed them in that direction, and following an inspirational visit to the ACAD, the hospitals trust realised that the TC programme gave them an opportunity to grasp that nettle and simultaneously increase capacity. So despite the initial reluctance, the eventual reorganisation of the hospitals included a controversial new TC at Pollford Hospital.

St Urban's, too, saw a TC as a way to help change patient flows (in its favour) across a wide part of the city, but unlike the previous examples they did not involve the PCTs properly in these discussions. The hospital simply assumed that once they had cleared their own waiting list they could easily exploit the gap in the market for PCTs around the conurbation that had insufficient local hospital capacity to bring down their waiting lists to meet targets. (In fact this turned out to be a fatal assumption; just over two years after it had opened, St Urban's TC was forced to close through lack of patients.)

As we shall see in Chapter Five, St Urban's was not the only hospital that failed to thoroughly analyse and think through its estimates of population need and likely demand for the new TC. Others also got it badly wrong. Ruckworth, for example, was partly designed to solve a pressing waiting list problem that was plaguing its host, a major teaching hospital, but it was also intended to reconfigure the services across the locality by providing a specialist service across several trusts for patients with routine surgical conditions who were otherwise quite well. The intention was to bring in large numbers of patients through the Patient Choice scheme, but in fact, within a year – by which time the number of beds had been increased fourfold – the flow of patients was only half what had been anticipated. This setback was partly because the planning assumptions about the type of case mix that the TC would attract had been completely wrong; rather than the majority of patients being minor routine surgical cases, 70 per cent turned out to be referred for major operations and/or to have other medical problems. The system had simply not been geared up for such a case load. Here too, the TC was destined not to survive.

In short, although the increased capacity for the local health economy was often a strong incentive to open a TC, it nearly always proved to be a false hope. Such inaccurate forecasting of the likely patient flows was partly caused by the haste required in putting together the bids to open a TC within the timescale of the TC programme, partly by the lack of good epidemiological information and analytic skills. But it was also partly because some of the planning teams were so enthusiastic to get the new facility and develop the new ways of delivering care that they turned a blind eye to the lack of supporting evidence about the viability of the likely patient flows and case mix. Major decisions seemed sometimes to rest on an almost cursory estimate of need that then became entrenched as a key part of the case for opening a TC. We shall have much more to say about this in Chapter Seven.

Improving kudos

Improving the profile of the organisation

For some idealists throughout the sample, the motivation to have a TC was simply to try to be among the best – for surely all the best hospitals would have a TC – but usually this was tinged with more pragmatic aims. Even sites that were less overtly entrepreneurial and ambitious than St Urban's, Ruckworth or Stanwick saw the potential for attracting patients from beyond their immediate area, so boosting the financial soundness and the local prowess of their trust. At Lakenfield, for example, having a TC was crucial to staying in the frame for the forthcoming regional rethink of service provision. And Brindlesham were in little doubt about the local political benefits that would accrue from opening a TC following the furore over the earlier hospital closure at that site. The chance of attracting patients from afar, while a welcome bonus, was a side issue compared to the chance of putting the hospital back on the map by providing an excellent new service that everyone would sit up and notice. Indeed many in the Brindlesham community regarded it not as a TC but as a replacement hospital.

At St Urban's where, as we have seen, the TC was perceived as a matter of increasing efficiency and productivity (quantity) at least as much as improving the patient experience (quality), it was also a way to remain politically ahead of the game. As a major teaching hospital, St Urban's needed to have the kudos of at least meeting the government's performance targets. Yet, embarrassingly, it was failing on many of them and the TC was potentially a way to help redress these weaknesses. Although St Urban's did have its share of influential modernising idealists, few among the senior staff believed that the rhetoric of modernisation was really driving the TC. What mattered was staying in the government's and media's 'good books' – such as by getting waiting lists down, improving financial viability and engaging in the spirit of the modernisation effort. By doing all of that, a TC was vital to maintaining the hospital's kudos.

Realising personal ambition or vision

It was not always easy to distinguish idealistic zeal from enthusiasm that owed more to corporate loyalty or even personal ambition. The three were often intermingled, especially as there was no shortage of personal kudos to be had from playing one's part in setting up a TC. Many of the early enthusiasts (often opportunists in more than one sense) made enviable career moves once the TC was established. At Brindlesham, for example, much of the TC's undoubted success was widely attributed to the project manager who was brought in as a champion of the concept, bringing with him experience and a clear vision to a project that until then had been fired mainly by the pragmatic and opportunist desire to replace lost local hospital services. His success in realising that vision made the TC, which was to become almost a hospital in its own right, a showcase for the TC programme as a whole as well as for the local SHA and region. It also gave him the opportunity to move on to a prestigious job in the private sector.

The sample sites included examples of 'turf battles' where, as is so often the case, it is difficult to distinguish whether the victories and defeats – which did so much to shape the configuration of the TCs – were personal, ideological or professional/'tribal'. The fundamental questions about the ways to improve care or throughput were often closely bound with personal reputations and power games. Sometimes, however, it was wider political forces that dictated a particular approach to thinking about the TC in the local context. For example, at Robbleswade the arguments over private financing that lingered on from the recent new hospital build (and followed through the TC build) left the management team caught between hostile trade unions and a government pressing for a success story in time for the election. Managing that situation was at least as much about retaining organisational and personal reputation as it was about modernising care.

Taking on the innovation: common threads

There were many reasons why a local trust would opt to take up the challenge of establishing a TC, reasons rooted in local history and context unique to each site. However, there were some common features.

First, the decision to open a TC was usually dependent on resolving conflicting views between different individuals or groups within organisations who were themselves subject to pressures from their local internal and external environment. It is clear that while initially there was a strong role for opportunists to get the idea off the ground, in the subsequent stages the particular version of a TC taken up by the organisation was developed out of the ongoing struggles between opportunists, idealists, pragmatists and sceptics. Idealists saw the TC as a chance to improve patient care, but there were nearly always sceptics who saw it at best as yet another fad, opportunists who wanted to grab the funding to develop a new service that was in any case much needed, and pragmatists who wanted to do whatever seemed most likely to improve the service with minimum fuss. Even where there was consensus among those with the power to make the final decision, there were always discrepancies about their underlying motivations, rationales and intended outcomes.

Second, they all had a genuine desire to improve their hospital in terms of quality, quantity and/or kudos. In improving quality some sites prioritised patient-focused approaches to care or modernising patient processes, but improvement in quality was also taken to include fundamental reforms of traditional clinical roles and practices and transformations in skill mix. In improving quantity they were hoping to increase capacity, throughput and activity, and in this they were tightly coupled to an agenda set down by the Department of Health, which (Chapter One) was chiefly concerned with reducing waiting times and increasing activity and efficiency. In improving kudos for the organisation, the sites were hoping their TC would give the organisation (and/or the individual senior managers) competitive advantage – or at least prevent them losing their edge or falling behind.

There is a tendency (which will become all too clear in Chapter Four) for policy makers at the centre of a large organisation like the NHS to believe that when a good innovation becomes policy it will, given sufficient incentives and/or funding, be simply taken up and implemented locally. Rather, what we have found is that this innovation was always reconstituted in a local form. This chapter has shown part of the reason why that is so. It is not that the idea of a TC was controversial; far from it. The concept of a TC had few detractors. Nor was it simply that each local trust had its own different reasons or capacity to set up a TC. Rather, there was always a shifting and varied configuration of views that led to an evolving and constantly negotiated clusters of decisions, fired by differing incentives, which gradually emerged as something approaching at least some of the initial visions of a TC. For this reason if no other, it was never the case that a hospital trust would simply take on the blueprint of a TC as put forward by some other agency – be it the Department of Health, a model TC such as the ACAD or even one local champion's vision – and bring it straightforwardly into being. It was never a clear-cut process of implementing a standard, existing innovation. As we shall see in Chapter Seven, organisational researchers and theorists (for example, Pettigrew, 1985; Kanter et al, 1992; Van de Ven et al, 1999; Helms-Mills, 2003) have described how innovations undertake their own journeys, changing and evolving as a wide range of organisational and other contingent forces mould them into their eventual shapes. TCs were no exception, but, as we shall now see, those forces were often to prove overwhelming.

Note

[1] We were reassured that other literature makes reference to similar groups. For example Traynor (1999) identifies four comparable groups in his analysis of managers in nursing.

FOUR

The impact of the wider policy context

> The public's top concern about the NHS is waiting for treatment. (DH, 2000a, para 12.1, p 101)

> The national Treatment Centre programme is entering a significant new phase of its development. The change provides a simpler name for the public and for patients at this key moment. It does not reflect any change in the core characteristics of schemes, or the overall objectives of the programme. From now on all national publicity will refer consistently to Treatment Centres. All the Independent Sector schemes will brand themselves Treatment Centres under contract. It would clearly help build consistency across the programme and help build public recognition and acceptance (especially with patient choice in mind) if the NHS schemes adopt the same name. (DH, 2003b)

The "war on waiting" had been at the core of the NHS policies of the Labour government since 1997 (Harrison and Appleby, 2005) and set the overall policy context for TCs during our period of research. *The NHS Plan* of 2000 marked a shift away from reducing the *number* of people waiting and onto the *time* they waited, by introducing new investments and targets along with a wide range of policies to help transform the way that elective care was provided. The new emphasis was on TCs, day surgery, the NHS Modernisation Agency, specialty programmes such as orthopaedics and ophthalmology (an early focus for TCs) and 'Patient Choice'. The government also supported the development of new services in community settings; it also set targets for increasing the overall number of hospital beds and introduced a star-rating system for trusts' overall performance in which five out of nine "key targets" were related to waiting. In 2004 the government announced a new target for the NHS, that by 2008 no one should wait longer than 18 weeks from referral by a GP to hospital treatment. The target was to be helped by extra capacity in the independent sector, which was beginning to become available and was set to increase. By early 2005, the government had agreed to £3 billion worth of contracts with the independent sector to overcome shortfalls in diagnostic capacity alone.

TCs (both in the NHS and in the independent sector) were set up not only to reduce waiting times but also as the main vehicles for parallel initiatives such as improvements to patient access and choice, which were part of the underlying drive to move away from the 'command economy' into a competitive, quasi-market economy (Harrison and Appleby, 2005). Moreover TCs were also linked with wider moves to reconfigure acute treatment services through electronic booking systems, shorter hospital stays, 'downsized' in-patient hospitals, redrawn boundaries between primary and secondary care and 're-engineered' delivery of care. These manifold objectives lay at the heart of the wider policy context in which the eight NHS TCs were operating during the period of study.

Government policy and treatment centres 2002-05

In April 2002, the publication of *Shifting the balance of power* (DH 2002a) confirmed the abolition of health authorities and regional offices, and the creation of PCTs. At the same time, 28 new SHAs replaced the former health authorities and had a strategic role in improving local health services. Immediately after their establishment the Department asked all SHAs to identify any anticipated gaps in the capacity needed to meet their 2005 waiting time targets. In the same month *Delivering The NHS Plan: Next steps on investment, next steps on reform* (DH, 2002b) referred directly to TCs as 'fast-track surgery centres' and also – while asking the new SHAs to estimate the likely private sector contribution – stated that up to 150,000 operations might be purchased from the independent sector. By October of that year, *Reforming NHS financial flows: Introducing payment by results* (DH, 2002c) laid out changes to how money moved round the NHS, and set up incentives for hospitals to behave more like businesses (see the section on Payment by Results, later in this chapter). Two months later came *Growing capacity: Independent sector Diagnosis and Treatment Centres* (DH, 2002d), providing the 'background and plans for diagnosis and treatment centres and highlight[ing] the role of the independent sector in the DTC programme'. This signalled the beginning of the first wave independent sector TC procurement exercise discussed in the following section.

In January 2005, the Department of Health published *Treatment Centres: Delivering faster, quality care and choice for NHS patients* (DH,

2005a). This update on progress explicitly tied TCs in to delivering the new target announced in *The NHS Improvement Plan* (DH, 2004) – the follow-up to *The NHS Plan* – of ensuring that by 2008 NHS patients wait no longer than 18 weeks from GP referral to treatment.

Independent sector treatment centres and the 'General Supplementary'

> 'Here we are, we've got six theatres, we've got five wards, three have been completely revamped, we've got this fabulous staff, we've got all these amazing facilities, and we've only got 20 patients in the building ... [the government] insist on pursuing this independent sector nonsense, and I think that's what we find so frustrating. I think from the government's point of view, they just say, we've just got to increase the capacity, we've made this commitment to an independent sector, 15% or 20%, or whatever, and everyone's work has got to go through the independent sector, and that's the promise we've made. Well, that's fine, but then you are going to lose some NHS treatment centres as a result, so they've got to decide somehow, how that's going to work, because you're not going to be able to have it every way.' (senior TC manager)

Independent sector TCs were just one part of a wider concordat with the private sector, first announced in *The NHS Plan* and published a few months later as *For the benefit of patients* (DH, 2000b). In December 2002 the Department published guidance for, and launched, the first wave of independent sector TCs (comprising a planned 177,000 procedures per annum over five years at a total cost £1.737 billion) to be focused on cataracts, orthopaedics and day case work. In May 2003 the government announced that just under eight per cent of the total hospital activity in the NHS should take place in the independent sector by the end of 2005. The first purely independent TC opened in October 2003 and the following May 2004 the Department announced two supplementary contracts with the private sector to focus on mainly orthopaedic procedures using a scheme known as 'G–Supp' (General Supplementary), worth £54 million, that enabled primary care practices to purchase operations from the private sector for NHS patients. G-Supp would therefore make it much easier for primary care practitioners to purchase operations from the independent TCs rather than NHS TCs. One year later, when one fixed and two mobile independent TCs were fully operational and interim services were being provided on three further sites, the earlier target for independent sector work by the year 2008 was doubled to 15 per cent by means of a second wave of independent TC procurement launched in March 2005. At a total cost of £2.5 billion, up to 250,000 elective procedures per annum over five years were now to be procured from that sector plus an additional 150,000 ad hoc procedures per year at a cost of £175-£200 million per annum for the 'extended choice network' (DH, 2006a). The declared aim was to keep the NHS secure, while opening up the range of choice, capacity, quality and service to significant improvement via independent sector provision (Reid, 2005, p 10). Both independent sector TCs and the use of overseas expertise and trained professionals were defended as offering an efficient and rapid way of helping the NHS to meet government targets on patient access that it would otherwise not have the capacity do (Stevens, 2005). As a bonus, such moves might help break what was seen as 'a monopoly cartel or a closed shop caused by a tight control of supply and an encouragement for huge demand' (House of Commons, 2004).

Attitudes to independent sector TCs were by now polarising and hardening. Far from wishing to enter into partnership, many staff in the NHS TCs began to show increasing hostility towards the independent TCs; they began to see them as privileged to such an extent by the government that they now threatened to undermine their own TC's long-term survival (Donnelly, 2005). This growing feeling of unease was further fuelled by Department of Health pronouncements to the effect that the second wave was also about introducing 'contestability', that is, making NHS hospitals compete with one another and with the private sector. The then Secretary of State for Health's response to those who claimed the increasing role of the independent sector was a form of 'privatisation by the back door' was to reframe the issues in the language of equality and fairness, while reiterating government commitment to the founding principles of the NHS. Nonetheless, many in the NHS felt threatened by what they saw as a redrawing of the boundaries between the public and private sector, and there were flare-ups such when an Oxfordshire PCT was refused the right to withdraw from a cataract surgery contract with an independent TC when the trust realised damage might be done to the viability of the NHS's Oxford eye hospital (Carvel, 2005).

From professional magazines like the influential *Health Services Journal* – which devoted a blistering first five pages of its 20 January 2005 issue to the topic – to attacks from the NHS Confederation, to critiques from the Royal College of Surgeons, to the British Medical

Association warning of the imminent destabilisation of NHS hospitals by independent TCs that were depriving hospitals of resources and patients[1] (citing, for example, the closure of an orthopaedic ward in Southampton because much of its work had been taken over by a Swedish-owned company based in Salisbury), it was clear that independent TCs were stirring up a hornet's nest that was given widespread coverage in the national press. Indeed, one commentator suggested that 'no other issue among the avalanche of reform which has hit the NHS in the last five years has caused such consternation among senior health service managers' (*Health Services Journal*, 2005, p 3). Advocates of independent sector TCs and the Patient Choice scheme (see later in this chapter) fought their corner, however, arguing that independent TCs would raise standards and improve both access and choice for patients. They pointed to excellent patient satisfaction ratings and to the value for money achieved by the bulk acquisition of private care that the NHS previously used to spend ad hoc for individual patients. Despite the rows, the inexorable top–down pressure to introduce independent TCs continued unabated.

One focus of the rows was the question of capacity. The Secretary of State claimed that independent TCs were necessary because there was insufficient provision within the NHS. 'The level of spare capacity in the NHS in England, for which I am responsible is ... about 9,000 places, I think', he told a Parliamentary Select Committee. 'Let us put it in perspective. That is out of seven million treatments in and out of the secondary [i.e. hospital] sector of the NHS' (quoted in House of Commons, 2004). That was not how it felt to some practitioners working in our TC study sites, who vehemently disagreed. Far from the government claims of a spare capacity of 0.1 per cent, they were concerned that "patients are not coming", that their TCs were "running on empty" and that the problem had been worsened since the opening up of the market to independent TCs. These TC managers were bitter, believing that the government had become the masters and they the victims of double-talk. Others were more resigned, simply accepting that such disparity between the view from the top and the view on the ground was how the NHS had always been run. Unquestionably, however, there was confusion and disagreement about the different versions of reality being presented about NHS capacity, and the TCs were caught at the centre of that problem.

Another grievance was (perceived) looser regulation that the Department introduced to encourage independent TCs to enter the healthcare market, which together with other incentives aimed at the private sector led to frequent complaints about the lack of "a level playing field". While independent TCs were guaranteed five-year contracts at above the market rate to encourage their involvement in the NHS, spare local NHS capacity had to be funded in the face of uncertainty about even short-term activity levels and funding.

By January 2006 21 independent sector TCs were open and had diagnosed or treated 250,000 patients; a further 11 were due to open over the following 18 months (DH, 2006a). The plan was for independent TCs to treat a further 145,000 NHS patients in 2006 – less than one per cent of the total NHS budget and only about 10 per cent of all elective procedures – and during that year they were performing 4 per cent of cataract procedures, 3.5 per cent hips and 4 per cent arthroscopies (Healthcare Commission, 2007). Then, just as our study was ending in May 2006, came the announcement that seven of the 24 planned local independent TCs (representing some £550 million of work per annum) were to be cancelled and the remaining 17 schemes to be delayed. In the event the 24 schemes were pegged back to 10, providing just under two per cent of total elective activity and unlikely ever to reach the original intended levels. To date there has been no systematic evaluation of the impact of independent TCs, despite the recommendations of the Healthcare Commission (2007) for systematic monitoring, but it appears that 'their contribution has not been a significant factor in the dramatic reduction in waiting times for elective procedures', although they *may* have helped by stimulating change within the NHS (Naylor and Gregory, 2009, p 5), which apparently did not include changes in clinical techniques (House of Commons Health Select Committee, 2006). They did, however, have 'a significant effect on the spot purchase price' although they were 'not necessarily more efficient than NHS Treatment Centres' and benefited greatly from the 'take or pay' element of their contract, which guaranteed income whether or not the agreed numbers of procedures were performed for the NHS (House of Commons Health Select Committee, 2006, p 4). An independent review of a Scottish pilot suggests that if the findings of that study were extrapolated to the rest of the UK, then – thanks to the highly advantageous contractual arrangements designed to attract private companies (Plumridge, 2008) – they may have cost the NHS up to £927 million for treatments that were paid for but not carried out (Pollock, 2009).

Patient Choice

The government was determined that NHS patients should be given a wider choice of where, when and how they were treated. The aim was for all NHS patients to be offered a choice of four or five alternative providers (including NHS and independent sector TCs) by the GP referring them to hospital (Reid, 2005), so that they could, if they wished, pick places with shorter waiting times. This, it was reasoned, would stimulate competition and reduce the number of people waiting too long for their procedures (Harrison and Appleby, 2005, p 29). 'Choice' was introduced as a pilot scheme for heart patients in 2002; the London Patient Choice Project began with cataract surgery in 2002 and was then extended in 2003 to cover other specialities such as orthopaedics, and ear, nose and throat surgery, and then piloted in other parts of England.

However, support for 'Choice' was neither unconditional nor universal (Bate and Robert, 2005, 2006; Burge et al, 2005).[2] Patients were not moving around the system as freely and easily as advocates of the market had hoped. A report by the National Audit Office found that the roll-out of 'e-booking' (which allows immediate electronic booking of patients' choices) was so slow that only 63 bookings had been made by the end of 2004 out of a workload that was intended eventually to involve millions of bookings. A national study suggested that top-down implementation and poor strategic planning appear to have led to many TCs being built in the wrong places (Damiani et al, 2005). There were also shortcomings within the systems themselves; for example, a number of our respondents described how they had failed to anticipate the practical difficulties they would encounter in moving patients between providers, because adequate information, financial and clinical systems did not exist, or had never been designed with this in mind. Poor financial and administrative mechanisms for facilitating the movement of patients around the system contributed further to the early inadequacies of the 'Choice' policy by slowing down the 'transfer' of patients between providers.

Payment by Results

To enable patient choice to apply nationally, the Department started in April 2003 to introduce a new system known as Payment by Results, which aimed to directly link a hospital's income to the amount of work it performed. The scheme became highly controversial. The initial focus was on non-emergency surgery for 15 procedures, including cataracts and hips, both areas where there were significant waiting lists, and both prominent in TCs. The aim had been to spread Payment by Results to elective, emergency and out-patient activity, but following a 'financial rebasing exercise', which all trusts had been asked to complete by the end of 2004, the NHS Director of Finance and Investment announced in January 2005 that the tariff would apply just to elective activity in 2005/06 and that Payment by Results non-elective activity and out-patients would only be brought on line in 2006/07. Many saw that last-minute move as an emergency measure to halt a process that could have triggered a crisis in PCT finances. This was largely because the Department had based the tariff on activity levels for emergency care in 2003/04, which had since increased. Then, more significantly, in early 2006, the Department had to withdraw the full 2006/07 national tariff only weeks after publication. The tariff was removed pending work to correct errors in the original calculations. These financial twists and turns in Payment by Results – to say nothing of the perception that the pricing favoured some regions over others – took some of our case study sites unawares, undermining their original financial assumptions and introducing uncertainty about the tariff that made financial forecasting problematic.

NHS Elect[3]

Faced by so many challenges in such a demanding and confusing policy environment, several NHS TCs formed an umbrella organisation to represent their interests, NHS Elect. There was a story that the intended name, NHS Elite, was countermanded, which even if untrue betrays how the group was perceived. NHS Elect promised much, enabling members to share specialist knowledge and expertise (including arranging visits to the US to view the surgicenter model), to provide patient information and marketing literature with a common 'brand' and image, to actively market spare TC capacity across the UK and to provide a common link with the Department and other national teams. It also offered a one-stop resource for information about the group of TCs it represented, including a price list for procedures offered by each site compared with the NHS's national Elective Spell Tariff (Timmins, 2003; NHS Elect, 2004). The underlying intention was to form a chain ('a franchise arrangement') in which members would work together and compete effectively with the emerging independent TC chains.

NHS Elect had a slow first year when, according to both its own managers and our case study site interviewees, it was not very successful at "actually delivering stuff on the ground". It was relaunched with a reaffirmation of commitment from the trust chief executives serving on the board as well as the establishment of a new medical advisory board. In return for £40,000 from each member organisation, it offered 'a draft blueprint for elective care within NHS TCs which includes around 40 recommendations or stipulations' based on a US surgicenter's best practice recommendations, which was then developed into models of care for 15 procedures with the main aim of standardising patient experience across its member TCs. NHS Elect also established best practice links (that is, knowledge sharing), provided foreign teams of doctors as needed and actively marketed the spare capacity available in the member TCs. One attraction was the help member TCs received in implementing "the practical day-to-day stuff", because, as one of the NHS Elect managers pointed out, "They've got just so much on their plates ... that they haven't got time to wade through [the Modernisation Agency's] 99-page 'Step Guide'.... When you're running a busy organisation you just don't have time to do that." By the end of 2005, NHS Elect had grown to cover 17 NHS TCs and had become part of the formal infrastructure of support provided by the Department's Short-Stay Elective Care Programme to the NHS, with the stated aims being to provide "a very practical bundle of support", which included a common experience for patients, core marketing and consultancy support to members, opportunities to innovate and spread good practice quickly, consultancy and accreditation services and new opportunities for collaboration as well as competition with the independent sector TCs. An important goal was to create a sense of identity for its members in the face of competition where, as one NHS Elect manager remarked:

> '... one of the advantages that the [independent sector] has is that they can create a corporate ethos so that everyone who works in their TC understands what the organisation is about. Within NHS Elect that's more difficult because they're not only part of a TC – although ... some of them don't even realise they are – but they are also part of [a] trust, they're also part of the NHS; they're part of [a] hospital. There are all sorts of different affiliations and incentives and drivers.'

The rising storm

The rapidly growing NHS TC programme was a well-received, uncontroversial and much needed organisational innovation. The policy environment for developing it, however, was highly complex, uncertain and subject to political impulse and apparent conflict between the national and local level, giving a distinctly, and as far as those at trust level were concerned unforgiving (some would say unforgivably) 'unreceptive context' (Greenhalgh et al, 2005) for innovation, modernisation and change. Local policy decisions sometimes conspired to undermine the ideals of the TC programme. As we showed in Chapter Two, there were often deep running policy tensions between the TC, its host organisation and the neighbouring PCTs and hospitals. For example, one senior manager berated the top-slicing of PCT budgets to fund an NHS TC at one of our sites:

> '[It] has drained I would say approaching £100 million from the sector, and I'm a chief exec of a PCT with a significant financial deficit. It's a great shame, all this, because certainly having an elective ... hospital could radically change things for the better ... both for the patients, for the staff, training – everything. So I think it's a real missed opportunity. I don't know whose decision it was. If it was a politician's decision, it's almost forgivable. If it was a senior manager's decision, it's outrageous because it has cost this sector £100 million.'

Such local rumblings were often an important part of the picture, but it was national policies that caused the greatest universal concern. The way that Patient Choice and Payment by Results were introduced certainly rocked the development of NHS TCs, but the largest looming cloud was the increasing involvement of independent sector TCs. NHS TC managers were unsure if the independent TCs were there simply as a stimulus to stir up the NHS and drive out inefficiencies or as a harbinger of a more fundamental restructuring of healthcare provision. Were they, in short, intended to fill short-term gaps in NHS capacity, or was the NHS now competing with them for its long-term future (Carvel, 2005)? The Department, for example, made clear that for both sectors 'once a competitive challenge is introduced it forces the existing provider to re-examine their processes to perform as well, or better than the new provider' (DH, 2006a). The perceived 'unlevel playing fields' favouring independent TCs coupled with the rushed policy of Patient Choice and the confusion and alleged inequities of Payment by Results were potentially leading to financial deficits and uncertainty among NHS TCs. The concerns are epitomised by two comments from senior NHS TC managers as the policies were unfolding:

> 'It's all very well saying you have flexibility and choice but that's the problem; you're left with an asset that has a huge overhead that you just can't meet. And that's the taxpayer footing the bill at the end of the day. You need to try and

generate a situation where people do have choice but where you don't have a facility like [TC] that's half empty. There must be a middle way. You could probably operate at 5% under capacity but not at 50%.'

'… there is an increasing realisation on the part of the policymakers that these [NHS TCs] were a vehicle for great innovation and change, and now the people who are left holding the baby are basically in a terrible position that is not largely of their making. These business cases were signed off. They were predicated on doing additional work in order to meet planned targets, and the fact is that that additional work is either going to the independent sector or that the money somehow isn't with the commissioners. The commissioning process is too fragmented to be able to support system-wide SHA facilities. And the response – which is the automatic response of NHS trusts during financial difficulty – is shut down, take out capacity. Let's reduce anything we don't have to do. Let's shrink … most of the places are not the exciting, innovative, energised places that they were. They are people who are struggling to keep their heads above water.'

The next chapters examine how our sites tried to avoid drowning in this unreceptive, unpredictable and uncertain environment of the policy deluge they were experiencing.

Notes

[1] In December 2005, 68 per cent of NHS clinical directors responding to a British Medical Association survey said that independent TCs had had a negative effect on the facilities provided by their trust (www.bmj.com, 7 January 2006, News extra).

[2] For a recent debate on NHS patient choice and competition, see Le Grand (2009) and the series of critical articles in the same issue of the journal to which his was a response. For a sociologically informed review of the development of the policy during the period covered by our study, see also Greener (2009).

[3] Data used in this section come from a series of interviews with senior managers in NHS Elect, unless otherwise stated.

FIVE

Achieving the goals? How and why the treatment centres evolved

For all the optimism that surrounded the opening of the eight TCs we were following, by 2006, when our three-year study ended, St Urban's had closed and Ruckworth was on the verge of doing so (see Table 2.1, Chapter Two). Three of the others (Robbleswade, Stanwick and Northendon) were in deep difficulties due to a paucity of patients and were in discussions about selling space and/or capacity to the independent sector. (Since then, however, they have resolved their problems in their different ways and are still, in 2010, operating as NHS TCs.[1]) Only three of the eight were functioning in 2006 comfortably within the NHS as part of the NHS TC programme. Two of these, Pollhaven and Lakenfield, were relatively small-scale initiatives that had been absorbed back into their host trusts, but were still attempting, with differing levels of success, to practise the ideals of re-engineered care pathways that separated elective and emergency care, increased activity and improved patient experience. Only one of the eight, Brindlesham, appeared in 2006 to have weathered the storm to emerge as a stand-alone unit that largely mimicked the early ACAD and exemplified key elements of the original policy model of what an NHS TC should be.

What were the reasons for the ways the TCs turned out at the end of our study? To a large extent the answer lay in the available capacity of the hospitals in a TC's catchment relative to the total number of patients. At one extreme, Ruckworth, Stanwick and St Urban's were opened in an environment where there were simply not enough patients to allow them to compete effectively in an era of Patient Choice, 'G-Supp' or independent sector TCs (see Chapter Four), and the effects were devastating. Lakenfield, at the other end of the spectrum, had a shortage of beds and therefore faced little threat from such policy shifts. At the other four TCs it took a great deal of wheeling and dealing, competitive marketing and collaboration with the commissioners and providers of healthcare to achieve a reasonable throughput of patients because the original planning assumptions had proven to be over-optimistic. The immediate question, therefore, is why the predictions of patient numbers had proven so unreliable.

Planning inadequacies

'It's a mess because the business case never stacked up in the first place, because nobody really understood where the activity was to come from. Assumptions were made that it was all going to come from Patient's Choice, or directly from originating trusts, or directly from GPs, but nobody actually went out there and did a proper market analysis to find out if that is actually what's going to happen.' (senior manager, St Urban's)

'If we took this capacity planning round and said, "Right, that's the baseline", you can guarantee that in two years time it will be something completely different. Or ... you can wait another two years and do nothing and then in two years that will be different again.' (senior manager, working on Phase II TC plans, Lakenfield)

Most of our sites struggled to predict accurately what their activity and/or case mix would be. They had to make broad assumptions based on patently unsound data and with very little informed debate even when the higher echelons of the NHS scrutinised the business cases. When interviewees described to us those early discussions they often illustrated where the planning figures came from by wetting their index finger in their mouth and then holding it aloft. St Urban's, for example, suffered from unrealisable planning assumptions that led within a year to a shortfall approaching 50 per cent. Ruckworth TC too was facing a deficit of over £10 million by 2004/05 and had become a severe financial liability for its host trust. It had expected to attract thousands of routine cases through Patient Choice, but instead, once the waiting list backlog had been cleared, found itself dealing with half the anticipated numbers – most of which were far more complex than the planned patient pathways allowed for. Ruckworth's frantic shift from in-patients to day cases, streamlining and other innovations on the hoof were now being driven not by idealist modernisation, but by the sheer opportunism of finding new markets and efficiencies simply to survive.

Stanwick had similar problems, some of which might have been predicted with a more careful analysis of the local healthcare needs, but the original model had been devised several years before the TC programme was launched and had not been adequately revisited or tested in the rush to obtain the funding to open the unit as part of that programme. The TC ran at around 65 per cent capacity until it eventually met its original monthly target of cases some 20 months after opening. Waiting lists fell dramatically as other TCs opened nearby in both the NHS and the independent sector, which again meant a fall in the available workload. Moreover, Stanwick TC proved to be more expensive than its competitors, due partly due to predictably high capital charges, rates and service costs, but also an unanticipated (although possibly foreseeable) shortage of qualified staff requiring the use of expensive agency staff to fill vacant posts.[2] The unanticipated extra costs of the TC were also partly attributable to the large overheads accruing from its associated high dependency care unit that was greatly under-used since − in contrast to Ruckworth, which found itself dealing with unexpectedly complex patients − Stanwick's case mix had been much more straightforward than had been planned for, so that the high dependency facilities committed to dealing with complicated cases were an under-used drain on resources. Moreover the plans for the routine patients were based on US lengths of stay not adhered to by the local doctors, which also added to the costs. This damaging cocktail of problems was compounded six months after the TC officially opened by the completely unexpected introduction of the 'G-Supp' scheme (see Chapter Four), which made it cheaper for local healthcare commissioners to send patients to the independent sector or to other trusts, which inevitably they did. These and other problems led to financial losses of over £4 million in the first year.

Robbleswade's plans suffered from a different kind of unexpected setback. Their business case relied heavily on activity from neighbouring PCTs that had not historically sent them patients but were now keen to use the TC because their local hospitals were unsatisfactory. Shortly before the TC was due to open, these PCTs revised their commissioning plans − not because of any dissatisfaction with Robbleswade but because their local hospital had now put its house in order. This was a huge blow for the TC as, surprisingly, no contingency had been made for such an eventuality. Pollhaven was another TC that underpinned its original business plan with inaccurate capacity planning assumptions. The team later employed to run the TC described them as "unrealistic or just plain wrong" − over-inflated by as much as 300 per cent, they claimed. The TC was soon running at between a quarter and a third of the expected throughput − soon after opening it was completely empty on some days − but it was able to adapt and increase the numbers steadily, although still well short of the original expectations. Meanwhile a financial shortfall in the host trust meant that the whole project had to be scaled down anyway. Even then they had to urgently commission an essential dedicated operating theatre that should have been included in the plans but was not. If it failed to open by the end of 2006, one manager told us, "we're stuffed". In the event, they just made it.

Brindlesham too found that they had been over-optimistic in assuming that patients would be referred by distant trusts that in reality had either not signed up to sending patients or had found more appropriate closer, cheaper, often independent sector, alternatives. As in Pollhaven, the team was able to adapt to the problem, in this case by successfully marketing with other distant commissioners through NHS Elect (see Chapter Four). Likewise Northendon soon found itself with spare capacity and under-utilised facilities and staff. This site had initially wanted a day case unit that would serve its local population, but had opportunistically expanded the scale of its plans to secure funding from the TC programme. However, demand "dried up", partly as the sending trusts engaged in their own "waiting list busting" and therefore had no need to use the TC, but also because patients proved less willing to travel than anticipated. Also, the clinicians at these distant trusts were extremely resistant to the idea of sending their patients to an unknown facility.[3]

In short, seven of our eight sites found themselves in difficulties because their initial assumptions about the likely numbers and/or case mix of patients turned out, for one reason or another, to have been over-optimistic or erroneous. It is striking how often and how badly so many of our case study sites got it wrong, and how much of the subsequent effort was spent in trying to rectify the consequent difficulties. The eighth, Lakenfield, was a very different kind of unit, integral with the host trust and acting as a capacitor to increase patient turnover across a whole surgical division desperately short of beds; excess capacity was therefore never part of their picture. Even at that site, however, the planning for the Phase II stand-alone TC involved major disagreements based on uncertainty about its eventual optimal size with little evidence to support either the larger or the smaller predictions. The project team simply had to proceed, not least because the survival of the trust as a whole might depend on this strategy and they could not afford to stall it. Yet they knew that there was huge uncertainty as the region struggled to reconfigure services across a number of hospitals, that the recently introduced Payment by Results (see Chapter Four) looked likely to have a major but as yet unquantifiable impact, and that the new requirement to treat 15 per cent of patients in the independent sector was also likely to deflect patients away from the Phase II TC.

So, why did the eventual course of the TCs' workload differ so dramatically from what had been assumed at the planning stage? Poor information and lack of predictive capability clearly had a huge impact, but it would be wrong solely to blame that for their shortfall in reaching their initial ideals, or for the failures and difficulties the TCs ran into as a result. Better planning would not necessarily have ensured that these TCs came closer to the original model, nor would it have resolved all of the problems. As we shall show, the evolution of the TCs was a highly contingent process subject to shifting grounds, serendipity and chance events, dependent on the interactions of context, history and relationships both within and between organisations. In this they differ little from a general pattern to be found in organisational innovations generally (see Chapter Seven). More specifically, we found several factors that had strong impacts on the evolution of the TCs:

- pressure (both from external demands and internal enthusiasm) to move fast at the bidding stage, with a tendency therefore to 'cut corners' in planning;
- changing circumstances and policy initiatives, not all of which were unpredictable, and the lack of adequate contingency plans;
- lack of support from external partners (including PCTs, SHAs, hospitals) who were not sufficiently engaged with the project or had conflicting priorities, and, linked to this, a lack of strategic planning across partners;
- inability to realise the ambition to draw in patients from distant sites – an aspect of 'market failure' (Bate and Robert, 2006);
- inadequate support from internal stakeholders (including clinicians and managers in the TC but also internal systems and contractors);
- ambivalent or even hostile relationships with the host trust.

Pressurised timescales

'Things happened so quickly in that we were waiting for a long time to find out how much money we were going to get, then all of a sudden a decision was made, and it's "OK, here you go, now open the DTC and make it work by Monday."' (senior manager, St Urban's)

'The conversation I had with [Department civil servant] was quite bizarre. He said, "I hear you can open a day case unit treatment centre quickly?" I said, "Oh yes, we've got the shell, we could do it." "How quickly could you do it?" "How quickly would you like it?" "Well, the Prime Minister wants it tomorrow to sort out [the local trust problem]. He wants all these two-year waits sorted in 18 months.'" (senior manager, Northendon)

Everyone in the NHS hierarchy felt the need to act quickly to hit government targets. The government and the Department wanted to demonstrate rapid modernisation; every region and SHA wanted to be at the forefront of establishing new TCs; host trusts needed to compete in a short timescale to grab the opportunity to acquire the additional capital funding, and their local idealists were eager to open the new facility as soon as possible. In the rapidly unfolding context of impossibly tight deadlines, the inevitably rushed job ignored (or more accurately, chose to ignore) the shakiness of many of the basic assumptions. The question perhaps is how to avoid the collusion and 'groupthink' (Janis, 1972) that accompanies an attractive-looking innovation in a pressurised environment. In retrospect it is easy to say that more slack in the system, especially in the early stages, would have made a difference, but given that it seemed everyone would gain from having a TC, it would have taken a very brave person at the time to slow things down and insist on more time for planning and reflection once the starting gun was fired. Moreover, even at Stanwick – where apart from some rushed opportunism in bidding to the TC programme the planning had been ongoing since the mid-1990s, albeit for a slightly different facility – the TC encountered uncertain workloads, low throughput and failure to adequately adapt to the changing context, which suggests that it is the quality of the planning, not the time spent on it, that matters.

The shifting ground of policies

The net effect of the private sector, independent and NHS treatment centres combined with the activity currently taking place in host trusts will result in a massive over capacity in the market. This is the biggest threat to [the trust's] survival. (Ruckworth internal report, 2004)

'I think this year we were probably only sent ... about 190 cases from Patient Choice and it really has fallen off big time, I mean we were doing several hundreds last year. So it's a big drop-off but it's obvious that, as the waiting list gets under what an individual perceives to be not unreasonable ... you get less take-up, and people are unwilling to travel and they're unwilling, certainly once they're in the system, to change consultant.' (senior manager, St Urban's)

'... as various versions of PbR [Payment by Results] have been issued from the centre ... our scenario has gone from almost euphoria to muted optimism to being downright pissed off.' (senior manager, Lakenfield)

'Even if we lock the doors, redeploy all the staff and have not another patient in here for the next seven years, it will cost ... because of the overheads and the leasing, and whatever. So, that's madness; so you've got to fill it, and I think they're right to bang on about it, because, as you say, I think it is this conflict of policy. The government has set these policies, and I can see the sense in setting them, but they clash regularly, and something's going to have to give.' (senior manager, Stanwick host trust)

The plethora of national policy initiatives made it much harder for TCs to develop as expected. This was not just a matter of competing priorities, which are a normal part of any senior manager's job (although we were often told that some did "take their eye off the [TC] ball" because some new initiative had loomed larger in their field of vision). The NHS had been going through a particularly intense period of change since *The NHS Plan* (NHS, 2000a), which itself had followed a long series of reorganisations (some called them 're-disorganisations') under the previous Conservative administration. The consequent 'battle weariness' or 'change fatigue' and the lack of continuity and corporate memory may have contributed to the failures in adequate planning and networking that might have helped to avoid the mistakes. But above all, many of the government's three parallel initiatives, independent sector TCs, Patient Choice and Payment by Results (Chapter Four), actually worked to undermine the success of TCs. The government push towards greater involvement of the private sector in the delivery of care for NHS patients and the independent TC programme in particular had huge implications for some NHS TCs. As a result partly of private competition, Ruckworth was described as a "failing business" that had to be sold to the private sector or be closed down. In 2005 Stanwick also entered into discussions about leasing the TC to the independent sector, a plan that the trust explicitly linked to the government policy of promoting private sector provision, increasing plurality of services, fostering entrepreneurial competition and breaking the perceived stranglehold of the medical profession. Here, as at Robbleswade, there was considerable opposition from pressure groups, local campaigners and trade unions who viewed the moves as "privatisation by stealth".

The business plans of over half our sample had relied on Patient Choice to bring in large numbers of patients who simply did not materialise. Ironically, this was partly because the apparent success of other waiting list reducing policies diminished the need for patients to travel to be treated. The low cross-boundary flow was also partly due to NHS administrative systems that were not easily able to support it, but above all perhaps, patients were less willing to travel than anticipated. There were many unresolved questions and much contradictory evidence in our sample about how the public and their GPs felt about travelling to a distant hospital for earlier treatment. (Some TCs were blaming their over-capacity on the reluctance of patients to travel, others were surviving because they were successfully drawing in distant patients, and one based its controversially large numbers of anticipated patients on the assumption that the fiercely loyal local working-class population would not wish to travel. One SHA manager claimed that only 12 patients out of the waiting list of 2,000 said they would actually go to another provider, yet figures from the local Patient Choice scheme claimed that over 60 per cent of nearly 20,000 patients who had been offered a choice had accepted the offer to go further afield for treatment.) Given such glaring disparities it is surprising that TCs – or the government for that matter – did not do more to test the real potential for the movement of patients. After all, that was a fundamental assumption on which much of the government's model of commissioning was based.[4] Or perhaps that was precisely why, given the intense pressures to follow that model, no one was brave enough to suggest testing it before going ahead.

The third policy strand, Payment by Results, represented both an opportunity and a threat to the TCs. For some, it was another challenge to their viability because the nationally determined levels of payment were continually changing, often working against them by undercutting their costs. However, the complexity of the proposed tariff coupled with a lack of understanding as to how the new financial system would work also meant that some TCs could potentially benefit from the new tariff payment system as their costs were below national tariffs (if, for example, they were in a small trust with lower than average staffing costs).

Unsupportive external partnerships

'I think [Ruckworth TC] could probably cover most of the electives for the sector.... Fantastic support for each consultant. Massive research base. Great patient outcomes. I hope in time that will be seen as a resource. But I don't know why it's not been perceived in that way. I think it's just been seen as the big future hospital trying to steal the work of the other hospitals, which I don't think was the intention.' (senior manager, Ruckworth, neighbouring trust)

We often found that other NHS organisations were not supportive of the TCs. Key failures in collaboration sometimes included:

- neighbouring trusts that were unwilling to relinquish significant numbers of their own patients;
- PCTs that chose to use alternative providers such as independent TCs (even the host PCTs were sometimes unsupportive);
- cost-based decisions to minimise the purchase of care for some low priority routine conditions that TCs carry out;
- SHAs without the authority to strategically coordinate the distribution of patients between different commissioners and providers.

Sometimes the TCs were let down by their potential partners because the TC had simply not put enough effort into wooing and involving them – even to the extent (Chapter Two) of seeming almost to deliberately antagonise key organisations. Ruckworth, for example, was frequently accused of having excluded the local health economy from its planning to the extent that neighbouring trusts felt threatened by it and became hostile (a feeling exacerbated by the top-sliced funding for the TC). This attitude made trusts much less inclined to send 'their' patients to a hospital that they saw as "predatory" and believed might undermine their own viability, or to help find a wider solution to the problem of over-capacity. Local trusts became unwilling to refer patients because they themselves were experiencing financial deficits that made it more attractive to use their own beds to treat patients from a particular specialty. Competing government initiatives such as Patient Choice and 'G-Supp' sometimes made it preferable to refer patients to the private sector. Such attitudes and actions left some NHS TCs floundering. St Urban's (Chapter Three) had done almost nothing to ensure that the neighbouring trusts and commissioners would send patients to them in preference to all of the other alternatives that were available. Perhaps their assumption was that their reputation would speak for itself, but if so, it seemed more to confirm their local reputation for arrogance. Moreover the trust's frank entrepreneurialism led the local health economy to regard it with suspicion, leading to a vicious cycle where the local PCTs and hospitals were reluctant to work with the TC, and the TC and its host hospital became increasingly suspicious that the nearby health economies were just looking after their own interests and sending only "rubbish patients".

Competition and market forces

'I tell you, the other day I found out and could not believe it that [nearby Hospital K] said that through the Patient Choice initiative there is money to send a certain number of their hip and knee patients overseas, which is just crazy. You know, we've got the capacity to do it, [Hospital L] has got the capacity to do it, I would imagine [Hospital M] have got the capacity to it – and you're sending them overseas!' (senior manager, St Urban's)

'We've been to the strategic health authority a hundred times to tell them that you've got to help to market-manage this: here is this facility, here are the waiting lists, this is what you are spending globally … this is bonkers!' (senior manager, Ruckworth)

'… the strategic health authority … have a real, real mindset of "Oh God, we're going to have [TCs] everywhere!" and in particular they're looking at this scheme and saying, "Well, do we really need it?"… It seems to have passed the strategic health authority by intellectually that we're a different business model these days. We're not going to be one big happy NHS family. We might have been in 1997 but policy is that we're competing organisations now and, not only that, we are much more fiercely competing organisations.' (senior manager, Lakenfield)

Sometimes the explanation for such activity was simple: market forces and the need to maximise efficiency. At Stanwick, for example, local PCTs inevitably leapt to take advantage of 'G-Supp' (see Chapter Four) to send patients to the private sector because that was less expensive than the TC. That, coupled with the pressure to make the best use of Patient Choice to reduce waiting lists, led to some perverse outcomes such as patients being sent to the private sector or even overseas for operations when these could have been accommodated in nearby under-used facilities. SHAs or local Patient Choice schemes might have mitigated that problem by brokering or 'regulating' activity, which did happen at some of the sites. For example, the local SHA eventually helped Ruckworth to obtain support to try and minimise the financial deficit, but the authority were limited in what they could achieve and the TC really needed much more support than was possible. SHAs were also undergoing organisational change in this period, and many were still finding their role in the NHS. While there were occasional instances of such authorities supporting the TCs (for example, pointing out the need for a TC project lead at Robbleswade), there was little evidence that they were able to provide effective strategic planning or assistance, especially when commissioning was not their responsibility but that of the PCTs.

St Urban's managers were particularly scathing of the SHA's impotence, and also felt victims of an unsympathetic Patient Choice scheme, but many commentators blamed the final demise of St Urban's TC on its own failure to link up collaboratively with the local health economy. It is by no means clear that greater collaboration – even had it been possible given the competitive cultural and economic climate in that part of the NHS – would have averted the eventual outcome, but it is difficult to escape the conclusion that a more collaborative approach from the initial planning onwards stage might have helped. The competitive attitude that contributed to the closure of the St Urban's TC was generally being encouraged as a necessary part of modern NHS management, however. The prevailing view at trust level – and this was true throughout the sample – was that every trust had to look out for its own future, rather than consider the needs of the whole of the local health economy.

Coordination and collaboration: primary care trusts and their strategic health authorities

'… working has become easier with the appointment of this deputy director of commissioning. When I started off she wasn't there so I feel like I've got a buddy on the other side now and that's just been really useful. We can just sit down and thrash it out and work out what we're going to do. It's very supportive and she's been good news.' (senior manager, Robbleswade)

Despite the over-riding competitive thrust, some TCs did manage to establish good relations with local organisations, especially PCTs, which often yielded dividends. Stanwick's good links with its main PCT – both personal and through formal committees –were important to ensuring appropriate patient flows. At Robbleswade and Stanwick some of the new ways of working (see Chapter Six) that revolved around shorter lengths of stay and more rehabilitation (in particular, physiotherapy for patients undergoing joint replacement) required working closely with the PCT managers and clinicians responsible for these aspects of care to allay their serious concerns about the dangers of patients going home too soon. However, the closeness could be a double-edged sword where, for example, PCT managers knew the trust managers well enough to observe what they saw as their failings.

At Brindlesham there were good links with local PCTs and the SHA because they had common cause in reinstating some kind of hospital facility at that site, and this helped the TC to attract patients. Some distant commissioners that the TC relied on were not accorded such close ties and had mixed feelings about the usefulness of the TC, eventually withdrawing the contract in favour of local, more extensive, cheaper provision that had been developed nearer home. Apart from that lapse, the key to Brindlesham's ultimate success was its ability to forge good links with potential partners that would supply it with patients – including the independent sector – and to be flexible in response to those partners' needs for changing types of facilities (for example, moving from day to short-stay surgery), all of which helped considerably in its financial profile and survival. When Robbleswade found that the contracts representing over half its proposed activity were withdrawn by two (of three) commissioning PCTs, the TC was likewise forced to rethink both activity and case mix. There was perhaps understandably considerable anger and bitterness directed at the two trusts concerned, a sense that there had been a breach of faith. However, a few key managers saw it as just another setback to be overcome, ideally by focusing on more positive relationships with the remaining PCT, and developing new links in the wider health economy. The latter entailed forging links with national networks as well as marketing the TC more effectively and more widely.

However carefully TCs tried to cultivate them, relationships sometimes became strained because of problems they could not have anticipated. For example, at Northendon, when it became clear that the

TC had over-performed for a PCT that was overspent and therefore unable to pay for the agreed extra work, relations became very tense and confrontational over the following year. The host trust began actively to market the TC capacity elsewhere with some limited success, but the legacy of this episode was a continued and significant financial deficit.

Nevertheless, in conclusion, it seemed that good, collaborative relations with the 'customers' (PCTs, trusts) and 'regulators' (SHAs, Patient Choice) could help to ensure an adequate flow of patients. Some TCs may have failed to attract the intended numbers of patients because they had not nurtured those relationships. More careful exploration (and perhaps 'warming up') of the likely market at the planning stage might have helped if only by alerting the TC to the possible knock-on effects of changes in the market. And when over-capacity loomed, the collaborative management of the market that may have been the best way forward were sometimes impossible because the necessary trusted relationships had not been cultivated. This in turn was at least partly attributable to two aspects of general NHS policy: the encouragement of competition and the lack of consistency and continuity of relationships that resulted from the frequent organisational upheavals. Whatever the reason for the lack of collaborative networks in some of our sites, and from whichever side the relationships' failures stemmed, the consequence was always detrimental to the TC as an organisational innovation.

Naturally the need to attract more patients in a competitive environment required the trust to sell itself through conventional marketing methods as well as through improving its organisational networks. Several interviewees (both external and internal to the TCs) emphasised the need to pay greater attention to marketing in order to ensure that PCTs, non-host trusts, GPs and the local population knew enough about the TC to want to select it as a preferred provider. Such marketing activity was not something that those working within the NHS had been used to and was not generally very intensive or sophisticated. In the main it was no more than leaflets, websites, local awareness raising campaigns and profile raising such as celebrity or royal grand openings. It was not possible to ascertain how much difference such relatively rudimentary marketing activities made, even for the TC that won a national NHS communications award for its efforts.

The right staff: recruiting and retaining key clinicians and managers

Another aspect of marketing was the need to attract good staff to work in the TC. Part of the architectural and technological design task for the Phase II TC at Lakenfield, for example, was to actively sell it as a really exciting and attractive place to work, stressing the innovative ways of working, the up-to-date equipment and the modern surroundings. Other TCs had a range of strategies that proved effective in attracting key staff who might otherwise have stayed away or been attracted by rival organisations, but some had more difficulty, such as Pollhaven, for whom the reluctance of the doctors to travel the short distance from one hospital to another remained an obstacle throughout. The rivalry between the trust's two hospitals was part of the problem, which, despite all the efforts of the senior clinical managers "just working quietly, subtly along the lines of digging heels out of the sand", left some consultants still refusing to work at the Pollford TC site. Things were different at Brindlesham where after some initial misgivings surgeons and anaesthetists from nearby hospitals began to see the attractions of doing sessions at the TC. This required a good deal of dedicated networking from a manager whose key job was to increase activity at the TC, but may also have been helped by the local politics being so strongly in favour of the survival of the TC hospital site.

Stanwick provides a final example of the importance of staffing. A board meeting there, reviewing the internal reasons for the TC's dire predicament, cited six main causes, of which three were connected with a failure to find staff who would be willing and able to undertake the new kinds of work expected. Attempts to recruit key staff were further complicated by the human resources (HR) procedures and policies of the host trust. Stanwick TC was wanting to recruit into innovative roles, such as "advanced nurse practitioners", but the host trust's HR department refused to recognise this role, forcing the TC to regrade the post according to existing staffing profiles, which made recruitment harder. Elsewhere the selective recruitment of key senior clinicians backfired on the TC's reputation because of what was seen as "favouritism", adding to the general hostility from neighbouring trusts. As all these examples show, the wider circumstances and local politics and attitudes often made it difficult to staff these innovative sites appropriately.

An organisational innovation such as a TC needed continuity of project management preferably from the planning stage, through recruiting and training staff, marketing the new service – one of the strengths, for example, that had helped the ACAD (see Chapter One) to deal with all the setbacks. Unfortunately, at a number of the TCs, the turnover of senior project managers was itself one of the setbacks that undermined them. At St Urban's, to take an extreme example, there were four changes of project leader between the opening and eventual closure of the TC – usually because the person concerned made a career move upwards on the basis, ironically, of their contribution to the TC. Not only did this lead to delays in setting up basic systems within the TC, but it meant that vital external links and relationships were never properly established. The host trust also saw senior executives moving on to other priorities, leaving a series of managers to grapple with the ominous problems that were eventually to kill the TC. At Stanwick, which had been jointly set up by several trusts, all the key local 'champions' had moved on and the TC managers complained of having to re-sell the TC concept all over again to the new chief executives of the partner trusts. At the other end of the spectrum, Lakenfield, which steadily increased its activity, efficiency, influence and impact on the improvement to the hospital's performance figures over the three years of our fieldwork, had no significant staff changes in the management. At Brindlesham, although there were three changes of chief executive of the host trust, which was in chronic financial difficulty, there was one TC project manager throughout who retained the authority to take charge of the entire setting up and running of this ultimately successful TC.

Connecting systems

'The technology hasn't caught up. So we're going to open a TC using old technology and then find it very difficult to implement new technology. It's always better when you're opening a brand spanking new thing like this, you might as well do the whole thing at once because people will accept it. It will be much harder to get them to change after. So that I think is a bit of a sadness that we've not quite got there because of the technology.' (senior manager, Pollhaven)

'One of the biggest problems that we've had from the beginning is that the hospital PAS [Patient Administration System] ... is not really set up to deal with varying trusts sending their patients and then us giving them information back as to what's happened to them in as much as information that they can then confidently take the next

> step with whatever they have to do with their patients....
> So we've got this terrible situation we've had for a year of
> balancing patients with two systems so that the quality of
> the data being put in is questionable when you've got two
> systems going on and we're managing patient information
> with spreadsheets.' (senior manager, Stanwick)

An innovation as complex as a TC, relying on a wide range of key actors,
including subcontractors, could only be expected to survive if active
steps were taken to ensure that all the relevant systems were properly
in place. This was by no means always successfully accomplished. Six of
the TCs we were studying had major problems with the information
systems on which their modernised care was expected to rely. Pollhaven's
computerised scheduling system, for example, made little progress,
particularly in relation to the interface with trust-wide and national
systems. Some of the blame lay also with an inadequate emphasis on
the development of the information technology per se, and some was
due to the failure to adequately connect the information technology
to the entire process redesign of patient pathways and staffing. At
Brindlesham an incompatibility between the existing digital imaging
service and the system to be installed in the new (stand-alone) hospital
site delayed progress for a while and ultimately required a different –
and more expensive – technical solution. Despite much early talk of
electronic records and digital imaging, Northendon also encountered
significant problems, notably in processing patients from outside the
trust catchment area, which led to apocryphal tales of patient notes
and X-rays being couriered by taxi "in carrier bags" from distant trusts.
Likewise at Stanwick the information systems were simply not geared
up to support the TC activity and at Robbleswade, despite it being
an ultra-modern new build, theatre scheduling lists were still being
prepared manually, aided by a variety of ad hoc individually developed
software solutions. St Urban's also ran into various information
technology difficulties but, typically, saw the blame as resting with the
other organisations with which the TC interacted.

Finally, in terms of internal relationships it should not be forgotten
that other agencies such as architects, builders, supply companies and
hospital support services such as central sterile supplies departments all
needed to play their parts as agreed, and when they failed to do so, the
innovation could and did suffer setbacks. Alongside these relationships
other factors, notably construction problems at the new-build sites and
failures in electrical and telephony services, provided further hiccups
in the developmental career of the TCs.

The parent trust – governance and autonomy

'It does [feel like an organisation by itself]. It does a little bit. I think in a way that that was bound to happen I think there's been confusion over clarity of roles, really. Are they being managed by the general manager here or are they managed by the Head of Radiology [in the host trust]? And that is quite difficult. I'm not sure the trust has got to grips with that yet. They're just evolving as things come up and that has been an issue with governance.' (senior manager, Brindlesham)

'... [The TC] was very much an independent republic and [now] it is much more seen as a divisional directive which has both strengths and weaknesses, strength in terms of corporate information.... The downside is that it is now being perceived as just another division of [parent trust] and clearly that is not the case.' (senior manager, Ruckworth)

TCs had to establish themselves as distinct and reputable entities not only with potential commissioners, patients and the higher echelons of the NHS and the Department – as well as their own staff – but also with the host trust. We saw in Chapter Two that the TC was often expected to solve the longstanding problems of the host trust. To what extent did they manage to do that and how did the relationships with hosts develop? It was difficult to avoid an analogy between the relationship of the TC with the trust and that between a recently matured offspring and its parents. There were interrelated tensions over:

- autonomy – the freedom to act independently from the parent
- finance – arguments over money
- help with a struggling 'family business'
- conflicting attitudes/ethos between parent and offspring
- parental pride in achievements that reflected well on them versus concern about failures that backfire on them
- the offspring's resentment when the parent took credit for their successes, but evaded responsibility for their failures.

The tensions depended partly on the character and standing of the 'parent', partly on the actions of the innovative offspring and partly on the material circumstances in which they both found themselves. These scenarios played out in a variety of ways. Brindlesham gradually increased its independence from the parent trust. The manager of the TC sat on the trust board (thus strengthening the links and visibility between the two), but the TC had its own clinical board and other structures that confirmed this semi-autonomous nature rather than being fully integrated within the trust. In general this degree of separateness was clear, but in the early stages there was some confusion not least as regards responsibility for the clinical governance of a facility that did things very differently from the rest of the trust, which was a challenge to be carefully overcome. Such uncertainty was quite common among sites where there was a degree of autonomy; the desire for entrepreneurial freedom clashed with the need for bureaucratic control of publicly funded services. Not only was there a question about accountability for public funds, but also for clinical governance. If the TC was allowed full autonomy, then was it also responsible if there was an untoward clinical event? Or would the host trust be held responsible, in which case could the trust not justifiably insist on keeping some control?

Although the Stanwick TC had been planned since the late 1990s, as late as March 2004 one partner trust refused to approve proposed governance arrangements. Discussions eventually led to increasing reintegration of the TC with the parent trust and the replacement of the TC chief executive with a general manager with less scope to act independently when faced with the host trust's "options for reducing the cost of providing the service [which] should be pursued aggressively". The TC had been brought back into line with usual NHS governance arrangements with a shift to single managerial and financial accountability through one 'parent' organisation.

Wherever the tensions of autonomy versus accountability had become a concern, the overall tendency was for TCs' wings to be clipped. Except at Lakenfield and Pollhaven, which had always intended to be integrated with their parent trusts (and seemed to benefit from that status), it is striking that in all of the other case study sites that had been promised autonomy, the trend was inexorably towards reining them in, normalising and re-absorbing them into the 'usual way of doing things' in the NHS. At Ruckworth, the original vision was for a virtually autonomous TC but its manager reported directly to the chief executive at the parent trust, which caused difficulties until the original TC manager and the clinical director left. The increasingly daunting financial liability arising from the TC's inability to carry out the expected activity meant inevitably that the host trust reasserted control. Within two years, and after a period of poor relationships and muddled responsibilities, Ruckworth's original 'entrepreneurial license' had been, as it were, revoked and the TC became closely integrated with the parent trust. Despite increased referrals as some of the local trusts softened their view in the light of positive experience, the situation continued to look bleak. The host trust continued desperately to try to persuade the SHA to step in and convince local PCTs to send more patients to the TC and to try and stave off having to sell it to the private sector. At Brindlesham, too, after the departure of the visionary project leader, the management was restructured and the TC was drawn back into the host trust. Robbleswade (reflecting its origins as an 'opportunity' to expand the new hospital) experienced a continuing tension between being a separate entity or an extension of the hospital. As the financial pressures caused by the loss of anticipated activity hit home, the scaled-down TC became more and more integral to the hospital, with few lingering signs of its innovations. But in Brindlesham, thanks to very different local politics and personalities, the reintegration of the TC as a high profile unit of the main hospital had the advantage of making the benefits of the new ways of working more widely visible, and thus helping to spread their adoption.

Northendon struggled from a very early stage to persuade the host trust to ring-fence the planned care beds, and in particular day case surgery beds. The TC began as a day case unit that was then incorporated into solutions to the wider problems of planned care; this meant taking in-patients. It soon became subsumed in a much larger section of the hospital devoted to planned care being carried out according to the new patient pathways. Thus the TC became the beneficiary rather than the leader of a flowering of innovations in care pathways across the trust. But although the trust agreed with the principle of a TC, it insisted that the high level of emergency in-patient admissions meant that they could not always actually keep the beds there free for planned day patients. Knowing that this would otherwise completely undermine its raison d'être, the TC dealt with that problem by making the doors too narrow to admit in-patient beds!

The danger of a TC's ideals being buried by the bigger problems facing the host trust was not lost on those trying to establish the Pollhaven TC, and their solution was to try as far as possible to keep themselves out of view, as it were, from the quarrelling parents and "deliver a service change without it becoming contaminated by the other politics". But this did not allow them to gain the autonomy they were hoping for. The quarrelling was one thing, but the even more pressing problem was money. The deficit of several million pounds that developed in the host trust meant that plans to recruit an operational manager for the TC had to be shelved as funding was removed and the TC continually had to ask permission to implement many of its essential features. At Ruckworth, Lakenfield and Robbleswade too it was financial deficits – whether in the parent trust or its TC – that led to a loss of the TC's autonomy as an innovation.

At St Urban's the TC finally reverted to being a department of the hospital and, as the external flow of patients dried to a trickle, focused on using the increasingly spare capacity to get the host trust's waiting lists down. This helped fill its beds for the short period before it closed, but by this time the lengths of stay on the TC were the same as the rest of the hospital. Staff, many of whom had not been committed to the ideals of the TC anyway, were relatively happy about the TC falling back into the main hospital like a wave sinking back into the sea. Stanwick staff were, in contrast, very unhappy about the host trust trying to wrest back control of the TC because of its mounting debts. Many felt that the TC's 'vision' had been eroded by the trust taking more and more control. The TC staff felt that they had lost their unique identity, and that the failure of the innovation was the parent trust's fault. In fact the host trust had given the TC more latitude for rather longer than the TC's massive financial shortfall might otherwise have merited because of the trust's acknowledgement that its TC offspring was widely seen as raising the trust's standing. Nevertheless some TC senior staff felt that the innovation had been doomed from the start because they could never break free of the parent trust's longstanding inability to meet the waiting time targets.

Summary

In summary, all of the TCs were subject to poor planning assumptions; the individuals trying to put the TC into operation found themselves unable to accurately predict important variables such as activity and case mix, partly due to poor data and partly because for most sites the time frame for this planning was highly compressed. Both the planning and the implementation of the innovation were highly contingent both on the shifting ground of the wider policy context (Chapter Four) and on crucial (and often unhelpful) relationships with the health service organisations around them (Chapter Two), where there was often an unsatisfactory tension between competitive and collaborative approaches that was only rarely resolved by appropriate coordination. The TCs also relied heavily on having the right clinical and managerial staff in place throughout, a difficulty that could perhaps have been better predicted and averted. Good relationships (and compatible administrative and information technology systems) with the host trust and other key partners both outwith and within the TC were also vital to the development of the TCs, but were often vitiated by financial crises and local politics.

Such factors made it difficult, sometimes impossible, to create and sustain the innovation as originally envisaged, but that does not necessarily mean that the TCs were unsuccessful. However troublesome the environment and whatever problems they ran into, all eight had at least some degree of success in helping their trusts meet targets in increased activity and throughput and the politically all-important reduction in waiting times.[5] In addition, as the next chapter will show, many of the sites were also highly innovative in developing new ways of working that led to improved clinical practice.

Notes

[1] Interestingly, as Table 2.1 in Chapter Two shows, some of the TCs were faring batter in 2010 than the 2006 picture indicated. This may suggest that major NHS innovations take many years to settle and become established, or it may reflect the continuing changes in the context of the NHS between 2006 and 2010, or both. Without further research, we are not in a position to say, and must confine our comments to the situation as it was at the end of our study.

[2] Mistaken assumptions about the costs and savings from changes in staffing levels also undermined the intended switch to a nurse-led service (see Chapter Six).

[3] Waiting lists are often seen as being 'owned' by the consultant who makes the decision to operate. These decision makers were often unhappy with their patients going elsewhere. In the most extreme example of this a consultant based at a trust engaged to send patients to Northendon wrote to his patients expressing concern.

[4] The failure to test that assumption is all the more surprising since such market-based mobility of patients flouted the long cherished NHS ethos of continuity of care and of the doctor–patient relationship.

[5] The waiting list decreased by almost 400,000 between 1997 and 2005. In October 2005 the waiting list fell below 800,000 for the first time since records began (DH Press Release 3/2/06, ref 2006/0049, 'NHS waiting will be history, says Hewitt').

SIX

Improving practice? Evidence of innovative ways of working

Whatever the eventual problems, all of the TCs in our sample had, more or less explicitly, a group of enthusiasts, mainly the 'idealists' (see Chapter Three), who generated the momentum and the energy to try to bring about innovations and improvements in care in the TCs. For them, the tumult of national policy changes and failing local business models was background noise as they strove to introduce practice innovations for their own TC, invariably meeting local resistance from one source or another even when other sites might regard the change as unexceptional. This chapter examines those innovations in care, including changes in both the structure, such as transformations in the physical environment and in staffing, and the process of care, such as the application of new clinical pathways.

Achieving targets: structure, process and outcome?

Despite the mixed motives for the innovation and all the difficulties that emerged once they were running, most of our case study TCs increased the throughput of patients and all were thought by the wider health economy to be important contributors to achieving not only waiting list targets, but also providing greater patient choice. For example, Ruckworth, for all its difficulties, was nevertheless helping its partner trusts to meet the government's stringent waiting list targets. As our fieldwork was ending, an option appraisal there, which included the suggestion that the unit be closed down, concluded that the TC should be kept open, and a number of suggestions were made to help limit (and share) the continuing financial losses. This was based on the view that over the coming two or three years there would still be a need for at least some of the beds to remain open in order to continue to meet those targets. Even St Urban's, which was eventually forced to close, was able to capitalise on its unused facilities to make a significant contribution to meeting its host hospital's waiting list targets. Ironically this was not due to its different ways of working; the average length of stay of patients going through the TC was no different from the rest of the hospital. Its beneficial impact on the waiting time targets was due to the very feature of the TC that eventually led to its closure: it had a lot of empty beds, and these could be used for a one-off, valedictory blitz on the main hospital waiting list.

Some TCs also saw the opportunity to work more closely with the private sector, through schemes – as in Brindlesham – to rent their under-used space to independent healthcare organisations or even (discussed but then not yet agreed at several of our other sites) to take the TC fully into the independent sector. For the parent trusts this was an additional benefit as, relatively effortlessly, it gave them the potential of benefiting financially from fulfilling another of the government's (controversial) targets, namely, that 15 per cent of all NHS patients should be treated in the private sector.

In contrast, Lakenfield was struggling with serious *under*-capacity and the innovation of the TC was deemed a success from the very start because it immediately provided the essential means for easing the crippling lack of beds. The TC was thus allowing the hospital at last to hit many of the targets that it had long been unable to achieve, such as increased activity, reduced lengths of stay, fewer cancelled operations and shorter 'trolley waits' in the A&E department. The TC was an innovation that functioned not only as a way of separating elective patients and shortening their lengths of stay, but also as a capacitor for the surgical division into which all short-stay patients could be placed just as soon as convenient. Not surprisingly, such a unit was almost never referred to as a TC. It was led by a dedicated and experienced nursing manager, assisted by a team of enthusiasts whom he trained both to run the ward and to organise bed management and theatre lists across the surgical division. By boxing and coxing with the full complement of beds in this way the team managed to achieve *over* 100 per cent bed occupancy for the whole hospital most of the time. This entailed a great deal of enthusiastic but relentless daily grind by the senior nurses in the TC team reviewing bed states, visiting wards and cajoling staff, very tightly controlling bed usage by using easy, friendly, trusted professional networks across the hospital and a great deal of tacit knowledge about surgical procedures, recovery and individual surgeons' idiosyncrasies.

It was not within our remit to judge objectively the changes achieved by the TCs. Nor were we able to say whether the changes in ways of working might have happened even if there had not been a TC (after all, such innovations as the separation of elective and emergency, patients, nurse-led pre-operative assessment, telephone pre-booking and pre-planned protocols are not exclusive to TCs). We were, however, able to reflect the views of staff on the front line of these improvements to practice, which they saw as being due to the TC. In general many of them, even the sceptics, saw TCs as bringing about real improvements in the way patients were treated, for example in better scheduling and throughput, or in the protocols of care that patients underwent. However, there were different perceptions of that change process, particularly in relation to the scale and degree of 'success' of the innovation. Even at the same site we would inevitably hear differing views of how much change had occurred. At St Urban's, for example, there appeared not to have been much change in staffing, nor in the attitudes of senior clinical (especially medical) staff. Nor had there been much progress in introducing formalised patient pathways for pre-operative assessment, admission and discharge; the new protocols had made little impact on lengths of stay for elective surgery and were widely ignored by the senior doctors, who continued to rely on long established procedures. Nevertheless, even here the introduction of the TC resulted in a marked fall in the waiting times for many operations, and one could see that nurse managers also made considerable strides in improving the patient experience before the unit was forced to close for lack of patients.

At Pollhaven, where the TC was still developing when we finished our fieldwork, a disillusioned service improvement manager, one of the idealists, told us that the TC had not done anything "really innovative". Yet our impression in comparing their achievements with some of the other case studies was that this site was much more in tune with the modernisation agenda than most, rescheduling and relocating elective care, introducing patient pathways, hiring visiting teams of overseas doctors who had helped reduce waiting times and spreading some of the new practices further across both of Pollhaven's hospitals. It was latterly the host trust's financial crisis that was holding them back by putting a halt to further expenditure around modernisation and/or redesign, and which – coupled with his idealism – had probably led to his pessimistic assessment. At Ruckworth too there was considerable clinical pathway development work, but (perhaps because of the failure to engage the surgeons, most of whom were employed elsewhere and worked as visiting specialists) managers were disappointed that there were relatively few innovations in the actual surgical care that was given. However, they admitted that this was difficult to judge because there was no benchmarking against which to compare other services or the parent hospitals' own previous activity.

This lack of objective benchmarking or evaluation was a striking omission from the TC programme as a whole. But then, it is notoriously difficult to interpret routine data in order to make such assessment reliably and there has always been a general lack of political will outside academia to evaluate NHS innovations objectively. The rushed, policy-driven competitive ethos described in Chapters Four and Five was inimical to the rigours and long timescales of scientific evaluation that includes patient outcomes. The overwhelming pressure on TC managers and their host hospitals was to quickly show their success and develop 'market share'. Stanwick, for example, in the face of some fierce opposition, claimed in a press release issued during a campaign in 2005 to justify the involvement of the private sector that:

> ... the innovative treatment and the high standard of care that [patients] receive at [Stanwick TC] will continue and further improve ... [Stanwick TC] is already a local centre of excellence. By allowing an independent provider to manage these services, [it] can become a world-wide centre of excellence. [Stanwick TC] will continue to treat at least the same volume of NHS patients and all local people will still have the choice to be treated at the centre.

Such hyperbole was clearly not based on an objective assessment and nor was it meant to be. No manager would have been brave enough to commission one while the TC remained in serious operational difficulties and had an uncertain future. Even if they had, the results would have come far too late for the decisive battle they were engaged in. Yet despite all the problems (see Chapter Five) of poor planning, over-capacity, financial setbacks and the evanescence of the principle of nurse-led care, at Stanwick there were indeed some clear innovations in the care that patients received. Whether any of this affected patient outcomes we cannot say, but the changes in structure and process (Donabedian, 2003) included a pre-operative assessment done by nurses via a questionnaire, a nurse-led clinical pathway about which patients were supposed to be fully informed before arriving at hospital, well-honed individual care pathways with key milestones (based albeit controversially on US models), case managers in charge of discharge planning, PCTs providing planned intermediate care, and considerable redesign of the workforce in order to accomplish these new ways of working.

On balance, the view from people working in and around the eight TCs was mixed, albeit broadly positive. Some saw (and were proud of) innovations they had introduced to the delivery of care. Others were frustrated at the incremental nature of change and had hoped for more radical transformations which they felt were yet to be realised.

Our sense as outsiders was that many of the changes were indeed incremental – 'first order' improvements rather than 'second order' transformations (Bartunek and Moch, 1987) – but that they certainly appeared to represent improvements to practice nonetheless. They may have represented small, often low-level changes to ways of working, adaptations and continuations of change processes already in train, often borrowed from elsewhere or developed within the host hospitals rather than the TC itself. But we should not ignore the fact that what may be minor improvements to an outsider may to the insider feel very much like local revolutions wrought within power struggles, and requiring guile and patience and a strong will.

Changing practice

It will come as no surprise that those responsible for developing the TCs needed to invest a good deal of effort in persuading senior staff – especially hospital consultants – to engage with the new ways of working. All the sites had 'idealists' whose main motivation was to improve, even transform, the patient experience. It was not possible to discern any pattern across the sample that any particular professional group such as managers, doctors, nurses or other clinicians had a preponderance of idealists. For example, although sceptical hospital consultants were often the main obstacle, many of the enthusiasts leading the change were themselves consultant doctors. To a less visible extent, this was also true of nurses and other clinicians and managers. Each profession had its share of 'sceptics', 'pragmatists', 'opportunists' and 'idealists'.

Success or failure in that improvement endeavour was dependent on the teams' abilities to make use of the usual features of good change management in clinical systems, including:

- appropriate use of personal networks among colleagues where there was mutual trust and respect;
- harnessing opinion leaders, especially senior respected clinicians;
- learning from and building on the experience of success locally and elsewhere;
- understanding and thinking through, in advance and at every subsequent stage, the motivators and barriers among key staff, and working specifically to deal with those;
- timing interactions carefully to optimise the chances of persuasion;
- empowering staff who were already keen to change (including novitiate 'idealists');

- introducing a management framework (for example, a 'modernisation lead') and resourced structure to facilitate change.

As an example, the group of enthusiasts at Lakenfield steadily overcame the scepticism among the consultant body to the redesign of patient pathways by skilfully deploying all of those strategies and activities. The TC team there achieved what were for them considerable innovations in the way clinicians practised, such as new booking systems, and alterations to a wide range of clinical processes, which were the key to improving the hospital's performance. This happened largely because a small group of like-minded and relatively junior innovators were trying to redesign the way things were done and were using the TC as a vehicle for driving forward this campaign of change. They did this through informal encouragement and example but also through formal methods such as 'process mapping' exercises in which they went out of their way to include clinical opinion leaders. The group was supported by being given organisational space and encouragement (but relatively little resource) by senior management, but they mainly relied on the use of subtle techniques, building on their internal networks and gradually pulling in more of the senior doctors as allies to create a groundswell for change. They succeeded partly because the hospital's performance targets and problems demanded it, partly because they were enthusiasts with well-honed interpersonal skills who wanted to improve things for patients and staff, and only coincidentally because of the TC. However, the new patient pathways that emerged from this process were also an essential part of the planning for the much later Phase II TC.

When it came to overall success or failure of the TC, obtaining clinical support often paled in comparison to the broader strategic challenges of patient flow, capacity and financial flows (see Chapter Five). Nevertheless, clinical opinion leaders were an important factor at all the sites. At Robbleswade, the reception given to the TC was strongly coloured by the leading clinicians' expectations (based on the recent local history) of the likely benefits and losses to their own practice, and they fell into two camps. Some feared "losing out yet again" in their attempts, which had failed during the recent hospital rebuild, to improve their own specialties' services and this rancour remained a "huge big can of worms" for the TC managers. Other specialties saw an opportunity to increase their bed numbers and operating lists and were therefore positive from the outset. Because there existed reasonably good relations between managers and consultant surgeons, they were all gradually brought on board to play an important role in developing a successful TC. At Brindlesham, senior clinicians ensured that the changes happened, but they themselves had been sold the idea by a project lead whose vision of the new TC commanded their respect. There seemed to be three reasons for this. First, the clinicians were fully behind his enthusiasm to make the TC a success that would not only replace but surpass the hospital that they believed should never have been closed. Second, the TC manager's vision was respected and shared because of his experience in a renowned centre elsewhere, and the proposed new pathways were easily endorsed not just because they were modelled on those at the ACAD (generally considered a flagship success) but because they looked familiar and sensible to the consultants. Third, the growing pride in the success of the new TC reinforced the staff's desire to conform to its methods of working. At Northendon, the success in innovating clinical practice may have occurred in part because of a release of pent-up desire for change that had been held back by lacklustre managers. The appointment of a group of middle and senior managers with a strong business ethos, and, later, the arrival of a new chief executive who had a more open, participative management style brought a focus on modernisation and allowed the flowering of innovative ideas among clinicians that had remained largely suppressed up until then, but which could now be centred on the TC.

In contrast, at Pollhaven there was no senior clinician willing to be identified with the proposed changes, partly because of the local politics of the split site. Indeed several consultants who opposed the change made their views widely known. Progress was therefore slow, and required careful tactics of individual persuasion, often with limited success because of a managerial infrastructure that was unsuited to dealing with the rivalries and suspicions underlying much of the resistance to change. Progress was even slower at Ruckworth, where managers faced with senior doctors who did not engage with the new ways of working were unable to make significant progress in implementing key aspects of the new pathways, such as pre-assessment and follow-up. This was largely because Ruckworth did not employ full-time consultant surgeons, but used surgeons from the neighbouring hospitals whose patients the TC intended to treat. This limited the chances of working closely with them to inculcate a new attitude to the process of care. Nor did it prove possible – although it was strongly advocated in at least one internal report – to enforce the clinical pathways by including them in the consultants' contracts. At St Urban's too, opinion leaders maintained their scepticism; even senior consultants who were expected to help lead the change were ambivalent and some were thought to be quietly working against it so as to preserve their 'fiefdoms' (a view that, even if it were not true, revealed the dysfunctional lack of trust). So there was little change and most doctors at all levels continued to feel threatened, unenthusiastic or even resistant to the TC.

In short, senior clinical support for innovative practice in TCs was crucial and the degree of success in engaging them depended on various local political and managerial contingencies, linked not only to the local motivating – and de-motivating – features of the TC and its host hospital, but also to the levels of mutual respect and the quality of the networks between managers and clinicians.

Changing patients' experience of care?

Physical surroundings

'… you often hear people walking through the door and they go, ooh, it's just like a private hospital…. People do say it's extremely friendly, they've really been impressed with the care – we ask everyone to complete a patient satisfaction questionnaire when they leave and it's always glowing…. And the other thing is it's really clean and that makes a big difference. I have never worked in a cleaner hospital and it's beautiful and the domestic staff take great pride, it seems to me.' (clinical manager, Ruckworth)

'It's more like walking into a modern library or modern building than a hospital which is great. All the clinical type areas are hidden behind that façade and it's great. The waiting areas for out-patients are very nice, very comfortable and very modern with the seating. It's not typical NHS and I think that's a good thing. We need to break the mould really of what the NHS currently looks like – fuddy-duddy.' (PCT senior manager, Brindlesham)

One immediate and visible difference was the purpose-built and patient-friendly architectural designs that several of our TCs introduced. Some of our sample sites, despite being part of the NHS, had all the external trappings of the private sector, and this made them attractive and popular with the patients who went there. At Stanwick and Robbleswade, for example, patients found themselves being treated in modernist new buildings and Ruckworth, originally built as a private hospital, had been refurbished to very high specifications. Brindlesham – a refurbishment of part of an existing hospital – quickly became a showcase for the TC programme, paraded nationally as the epitome of the TC concept (see Chapter One and Appendix 1). Modelled largely on the pioneering ACAD (see Chapter One), it was housed in similarly splendid and functional new premises. Leather sofas and low tables furnished the burnt orange waiting areas, pale limestone tiles clad the toilet walls and floors and light streamed through a glass ceiling, creating a calm and airy atmosphere. Robbleswade placed a good deal of emphasis on the modern, clean, state-of-the-art look and feel of the TC, seeking to match the existing hospital, which had recently been built as a PFI. One difficulty arising from adopting the same look and feel, however, was that many inside and outside the trust saw this as confirmation that the TC was merely an extension of the newly built hospital, offering nothing more than extra capacity.

In contrast, at Lakenfield, where the TC was almost never described as such and was housed in accommodation within the main hospital, it was doubtful whether patients were aware of being in a different unit, as it was simply a modestly refurbished in-patient ward. There was nothing here to distinguish the ward from the rest of the hospital; it retained its old-fashioned, slightly worn, 'lived in' look. This was in keeping with its function since the ward was used not only for patients who came in for a wide range of routine surgery but also as a flexible space for patients (known colloquially as the "end of stays") who no longer needed to be on the main wards. Indeed for many patients, the only effect of being on the TC that they might notice would be that they were moved to and from other surgical wards as their condition changed. But the plans for the new-build Phase II TC (eventually opened several years later) were driven by a different vision that would also have the 'wow factor' whereby as one senior manager put it: "It's not [as in Phase I] just the efficiency gain with modernisation, it's the efficiency gain with modernisation *plus* 'God, isn't this a nice place' as well. That's what patients are interested in."

Innovations in patient pathways

'There is a definite sense that things are changing and moving.... [B] who was the waiting list manager, she said the changes had been quite staggering.' (senior manager, Northendon:)

'If I'm really honest, we're not always as innovative as we like to think we are … that's the sort of stuff that's going

on elsewhere in the country, so it's not groundbreaking.'
(clinical manager, Ruckworth)

Most of the changes described to us were not new; the ideas and methods were usually borrowed and adapted from elsewhere or occasionally from the Modernisation Agency's guidance.[1] TCs were, in other words, a form of innovation that was more *exploitative* of existing ideas rather than *explorative* for new ones. Indeed even at any given site, the new procedures may not have originated in the TC but elsewhere in the host hospital. At Robbleswade, for example, teams led mainly by nurses who were keen innovators ('idealists') were developing new patient pathways in the TC and rolling them out to the rest of the hospital but this work had already been well under way before the TC was even considered and there had been nurse led pre-assessment clinics for nearly four years in their host hospital. TCs were not necessarily *creating* or originating innovation, but acting as a prototype and field-testing site, which could be equally valuable especially when – as at Robbleswade – the use of these innovations was as a catalyst for change in the wider hospital.

The modernising efforts usually resulted in changes that included:

- the booking system;
- the pre-operative assessment;
- admissions procedures;
- new 'pathways' – remodelling the configuration of clinical investigations and procedures the patient undergoes;
- improved discharge planning and follow-up.

The director of Brindlesham, regarded widely as a model TC, consistently emphasised the redesign of working practices not only to provide better care for patients, but also, thereby, to meet waiting time initiatives, attract and keep staff and also attract patients from beyond the local health economy to raise its profile (and income), and also to spread the word about its innovative design and ways of working. An early innovation there included the design of administrative pathways for patients that gave a smoother flow from referral through booking and scheduling to treatment. This required the creation of generic clerical workers to support its implementation and was later used to support the clinical pathways in Brindlesham's contract with the independent sector and also produced a model of care that was later taken up by a hospital in Scotland.

Such changes appeared at all the sites to a greater or lesser extent. Unlike the traditional unplanned, short notice summons of patients from the waiting list, admissions were booked by agreement with the patient well in advance, sometimes using new electronic booking systems, taking note not only of the patient's condition but also their availability and convenience. Pre-operative assessment was increasingly carried out by trained nurses according to clear protocols, and including in some cases a home assessment questionnaire which the patient completed and returned by post before attending for pre-operative assessment. The patients' journey from pre-assessment through their treatment to discharge and follow-up typically followed newly developed protocols. These protocols were generally designed to streamline care; they would try to minimise, for example, unnecessary delays between different stages of the investigation and treatment, and to reduce the number of different clinicians and others that the patient came into contact with. At Northendon, processes from pre-admission through to post-operative care were thoroughly overhauled and modernised with changes – in the vanguard of those advocated by the Modernisation Agency – that were applied to a whole elective care unit (including a new surgical assessment unit) of which the TC was now a part. They included:

- telephone pre-operative assessment by nurses;
- changes in skill mix (including new assistant practitioner and anaesthetic practitioner roles);
- new operating theatre procedures including a linen-free environment;
- clinical pathways reducing length of stay (for example, knee replacements in four or five days, hip prosthesis in three days); these were imported largely from the ACAD when a new senior nurse arrived who had worked there and began working with clinicians to adapt them for local use;
- music in the recovery room;
- a discharge lounge.

At most of the sites, the patient's discharge from the TC would be decided (usually by a nurse rather than – as is traditional – by a doctor) on the basis of protocols that had been agreed for that particular condition. Follow-up would depend on clinical need (and not as so often in the past, on the weekly ward routine or the need to manipulate bed vacancies) and perhaps be carried out by community staff working to agreed arrangements, or perhaps, for example, by a routine telephone call from the ward to the patient's home. Finally, changes also included making more efficient use of existing facilities such as extending the standard working day in theatres (including weekends for elective work) to increase the throughput, or moving patients between beds, trolleys and waiting or recovery areas in order to free up the space for other patients in the wider hospital system. Many of these changes involved the agreement of clinicians to carry out surgery in different ways, such as doing hernias as day cases, or using local anaesthetics for more operations. As staff became used to the new methods, the list of procedures amenable to such an approach tended to grow. This was so at Lakenfield, for example, where more and more surgeons were persuaded of the benefits of working according to the new principles, such that the capacity of the ward had to be expanded by the addition of a pre-operative assessment unit to make the whole process of surgical admissions more efficient. They then began to move some of the more complex day surgery to that unit, all of which was designed to make this short-stay ward even more efficient as a way of dealing with the majority of routine surgery.

Usually the tensions between the 'idealists' and the 'sceptics' and 'pragmatists' ensured that many sites not only experienced, as we have seen, mixed success but also ambivalence in the very introduction of the changes expected by the 'modernisation agenda'. At Robbleswade, for example, as the TC was increasingly constrained by the wider financial and political problems of the host hospital, one of the 'idealists' was still required by the host hospital to work on a programme of redesigning pathways and staffing but was continually frustrated by the naysayers, especially given the TC's now very small size and diminishing influence. Stanwick was committed to introducing new pathways modelled on its US 'mentor' organisation, but the enthusiasm for the advanced nurse practitioner role, which underpinned such elements of the pathways such as pre-admission and ward cover, ran into the buffers with the senior doctors who opposed the very existence of such a role. St Urban's attempts at innovative patient pathways were dismissed by many of the consultants as unsafe or unworkable (despite the success of similar pathways elsewhere in the country) on the grounds that very few patients fitted the "bureaucratic template". At other sites similar views were not sufficient to block the innovations. A senior surgeon/manager at Lakenfield, for example, had started out as a fierce TC sceptic but on retirement had been persuaded to do a number of day surgery lists. Progressively he became a 'pragmatist' convert and a stalwart of the new pathways, helping to develop a pathway for hernia repairs. Although he was keen to point to the limited scope of the change (which he felt was "more or less a transcription of what happens anyway really.

It's a little bit streamlined, speeded up.... But if the patient doesn't fit the first box, nobody's interested"), he was nevertheless pivotal as an opinion leader whose conversion helped persuade other consultants.

An example at Pollhaven showed how the persistence of the local politics and rivalries between the two hospital sites affected a redesigned booking system. By blocking a change that took the waiting list out of the surgeons' control, the consultant body had potential wrecking power for the TC and could use clinical arguments that the managers were too deferential to counter despite considerable scepticism about some of the consultants' motives. Eventually they arrived at a pragmatically negotiated solution (a clinically trained scheduling manager) to allow the innovation to move on. It was the kind of tussle that will be familiar to anyone who has ever worked in a senior capacity in any hospital anywhere. Organisational innovation is not immune from, and indeed intimately relies on, the sheer mundane familiarity of contested, negotiated order that is part of any organised collective activity.

Our study was not just interested in describing innovations in practice such as the new patient pathways, but also in understanding how TC staff used different kinds of knowledge (evidence) and experience to develop them. Some of these pathways were borrowed from external sources where others had already pioneered new ways of working. Thus at Brindlesham, the consultants accepted patient pathways developed for use at the ACAD, which were trusted as having good provenance and championed by the TC manager whom they also respected and trusted. The fact that the new pathways corresponded with the clinicians' own views of good practice also ensured that there was little resistance to their incorporation in the routines of the TC. Many other sites, however, felt the need to develop their own pathways. At Robbleswade, for example, nursing staff initially expended considerable effort to dissect current practice for each procedure and reassemble it in ways that improved the patient experience and streamlined care delivery. About six months before the opening date for the TC, however, they decided to use generic pathways as progress was too slow. Lakenfield, however, persisted in redesigning their own pathways because the process of doing so was a cornerstone of their strategy for engaging clinicians and getting their ownership of the new ways of working. The evidence for their pathways was largely based either on their own experience or that of respected colleagues elsewhere (and a reliance on such colleagues being knowledgeable about best practice either through contacts or through the journals) and occasionally on other sources such as journals, websites and professional associations.

There appeared, however, to be little overt checking that the pathways conformed to the conventions of evidence-based practice. They, like other sites, had a much more pragmatic approach that melded many different types of evidence from a wide range of what they regarded as trusted sources (Gabbay and le May, 2011).

Innovations in staffing

'… here, at the brand new centre, it's just a real opportunity to be able to do so much more. We've been fighting for professional status for so long and to be able to take over what the doctors are doing and to be at the forefront, delivering what nurses haven't done before – we've got fantastic nurses. And if you go speak to any new advanced practitioners out here, they've also got the bug and they just think it's great.' (nurse manager, Stanwick)

'The place has been staffed in a very traditional way. I would describe the nursing skill mix as very top heavy…. And why it's happened that way I think it's just happened that way, I don't think anybody's given it an awful lot of thought to be honest.' (senior manager, St Urban's)

Many of the new pathways required changes in clinical roles that entailed breaking down some of the traditional distinctions between existing professional groups. Ruckworth, for instance, blurred professional boundaries with nurses trained to do post-operative physiotherapy and therapists trained to review GP referral letters in order to triage and investigate patients and decide if they were appropriate for the consultant to see. Brindlesham, like others elsewhere, developed pre-operative specialist practitioners with responsibility for pre-assessment, and also introduced advanced theatre practices by using two theatre practitioners (one a nurse and one an operating department assistant) to undertake minor procedures such as taking prostate biopsies. They also introduced more flexible use of skills such as using nurses to rotate through theatres, recovery and the short-stay areas, which made much more sense given the peaks and troughs of the need for different kinds as patients progressed through the day of their operation. That such changes were remarkably hard won was not just because of professional resistance. At Lakenfield, for example, the hospital set about introducing a new grade of healthcare assistant that combined the roles of a relatively junior nurse and an operating department assistant.

By allowing either profession to train for this attractive new role they would not only create a more suitable type of person for the required job, but ease their recruitment problems. Yet even though this simple idea had everyone's agreement and the TC could not be maintained or developed without it, the introduction of the new grade required very detailed operational manoeuvrings through broader schemes to recruit more nurses, to revamp the qualifications ladder from school leavers through to qualified nurses, to develop new curricula and assessments, to introduce new gradings and salary scales linked attractively to other career ladders, and so on and on – and all this in the broader context of economic and demographic trends that were impeding recruitment to the healthcare professions at every level. It was therefore not surprising that Lakenfield's other more ambitious (and contentious) ideas such as the introduction of non-medical anaesthetic assistants were held in abeyance until there was more evidence of success elsewhere in the NHS and the local doctors might be more receptive to the idea.

The shortage of suitable personnel often included surgeons. Two of our sample sites had overseas surgical teams flown in to do regular operating lists, and succeeded in attracting highly qualified surgeons from abroad. At Northendon this seemed to produce constructive mutual learning with overseas surgeons interested in sharing knowledge and techniques, but also learning from their NHS counterparts. While viewed positively from within the hospital, the arrangement was not without its critics; at least one surgeon from further afield objected on principle to having patients sent from 'his' waiting list to a distant unit to be operated on by "foreign" surgeons. Pollhaven had already used overseas teams before the TC opened, and found that the experience helped persuade some sceptics to see the relative advantages of 'factory'-type surgery. The successful experience of having foreign doctors not only provided evidence that the hospital could take on innovative projects, but also useful lessons about the need for continuity of care when designing the TC.

Planned staffing innovations did not always come about. Sometimes, as at St Urban's, they were stifled at birth by a variety of factors including scepticism and resistance or an insufficient drive for change from interested professional groups, which was a serious block to the innovation. In contrast, Stanwick's pioneering plans to be a nurse-led facility, a novel focus of the TC's original plans, were eventually enthusiastically endorsed by all groups including most consultants. Unfortunately the concomitant extra funds were not. Stanwick had initially trained some 20 'advanced nurse practitioners' who were intended not only to push the frontiers of nursing practice forward, but also to have an educative role in developing other key staff such as therapists and healthcare assistants. The rationale was to use fewer junior doctors,[2] resulting in savings from which the new nursing grades could be resourced. However, as the financial crisis set in (see Chapter Five) these rather loose calculations were superseded by the need to encourage senior doctors to use the TC. The funds saved by consequently employing fewer junior doctors were spent on paying those senior doctors, not on developing new grades of senior nurses, which came as a heavy blow for the pioneering nurses.

Different ('can do') mentality

'It's exciting! We're not standing still. There's lots going for it and there's a great future. And I see it expanding greatly. I think that is very good for us, the people, and everybody.' (theatre manager, Brindlesham)

'I say we're special because we give [patients] information, what they want, where other clinics don't. They're "Next! Sit down! Wait for your number!" But we don't do this.... We do a little bit extra than we need to do.... I chat to my patients, I don't just make it a formal interview. It keeps them calm and relaxed and they enjoy the experience, and that's what we want. We want a DTC clinic to be an enjoyable experience.... We sort out the social problems here. I had a case yesterday where I had to sort out this 80-year-old in a wheelchair who lives on the fourth floor in a flat without a lift. He's come for a knee replacement. Surgeon comes to me and says can you sort this out for me? I had to sort out the housing scheme ... you see that's part of my extended role.' (TC senior nurse, St Urban's)

'We had been trying to transfer a patient and the main ward wasn't able to take him. "What's the hold up?" we said. "We haven't got a bed made up", they said. "Right we'll come and make the bed for you" which we went up and did straight away and that way everybody's happy.' (TC senior nurse, Lakenfield)

An intangible innovation was the way many front-line TC staff did cultivate a different, and very distinctive, ethos from the rest of the hospital. At Lakenfield, for example, staff were clearly focused on getting patients through the system efficiently, and fiercely proud of their reputation for innovation and flexibility. Although this TC was integrated with the rest of the hospital, its innovative ways of working coexisted comfortably with the more traditional attitudes elsewhere in a trust that, according to TC staff, lacked the 'can do' mentality that underpinned the TC's esprit de corps, and which the TC staff tried to ensure was understood and appreciated by the rest of the hospital. This kind of ethos often engendered a collective feeling of almost euphoric pioneering spirit among front-line TC staff, which ultimately linked to much greater – and real, not rhetorical – 'patient-focused care'. There were also examples where management staff found that the development of the TC was also central to their own personal or career development, nowhere more so than at Northendon where the project to get the TC off the ground represented a unique opportunity for some relatively junior staff to develop project management skills that required a remarkable degree of 'can do', indeed 'derring do', mentality, exemplified by a middle manager who revelled in telling us, as her team rushed to open the TC on time, "No one else will help you deliver – you have to do it yourself." We were in no position to determine how far such individuals self-selected to work in TCs, or gained them by working there, but either way, TCs did provide them with important developmental opportunities. Indeed, with only one exception who felt overworked and rushed, we did not find examples of disillusionment or defeatism in any of the TCs' staff.

The struggle for a glass half full

'Here I think that there are certain things that we now take for granted, as normal practice if you like, whereas when I go to other places, they go "Ooh, that's a good idea!" and I think, "Oh? That's really basic to us...." So I think we are still innovative. I don't think, if I'm really honest, we're always as innovative as we like to think we are.... But having said that, we're making a lot of changes, in terms of day surgery, getting regional blocks, and sending patients home without any alarms, and so there is a lot changing, but it's *changing*, it hasn't necessarily *changed*.' (clinical manager, Ruckworth)

In chronicling the changes that were achieved in the face of the often formidable challenges that local managers struggled to overcome, one begins to put the scale and scope of an innovation such as the TCs into perspective. The task is made no easier by the lack of objective measures of success other than the policy-led targets that TCs were being judged by, such as throughputs and waiting times. Any judgement of the qualitative change, the extent to which the 'modernisation agenda' was achieved must rely on our informants, whose subjective views were coloured not only by their being, say, idealists, pragmatists or sceptics, but also the expectations against which they were explicitly judging their TCs' endeavours. This was illustrated, for example, by a specialist day surgery manager who was brought from overseas to manage one of the TCs and who struggled with a moderate degree of success to increase day surgery to levels that would be quite normal at many sites in the UK and further afield. He felt frustrated, yet locally this was regarded as almost revolutionary, and had been a real tussle to accomplish. Moreover, to observers the changes we have described may appear fairly small-scale and un-dramatic ("Durr!" a modern patient might say, "*of course* you should plan the management of an elective operation in advance!"), but when viewing the case studies from where the innovators themselves were sitting we could appreciate just how revolutionary and hard-won such an innovation could be. It is important for outsiders not to underestimate what was achieved, even where the local innovation might only be to establish practices that elsewhere might be regarded as standard procedure.

Notes

[1] The Modernisation Agency ran a series of 'learning events' (which resembled fairly formal conferences), typically showcasing what leading TCs were doing and providing an additional mechanism for disseminating ideas, alongside their various websites and Modernisation Agency publications.

[2] The lack of junior doctors in TCs (where operations were usually done only by experienced surgeons) led to debate nationally about the adverse effect of TCs on training. Professional bodies such as the British Medical Association argued that the removal of routine work from the mainstream of hospital activity would diminish the training offered to junior surgeons, for example by removing the less complicated procedures on which junior trainees might learn their craft. Not all our case study sites agreed – for example, Robbleswade welcomed the TC as a chance to promote training – but generally this problem was not mentioned at all. Subsequently, however, in response to these concerns – which the House of Commons Health Select Committee (2006, p 4) regarded as 'well-founded'– the contracts for Phase II independent TCs required them to make at least one third of activity available to provide training as required by the local educational bodies (Naylor and Gregory, 2009).

SEVEN

Summary and conclusions: making sense of what happened

In this chapter we begin by summarising our findings. We than consider some of their implications in terms of organisational theory before, in the final chapter, drawing out some practical conclusions and lessons.

Summary

When *The NHS Plan* was launched in 2000, TCs were a promising organisational innovation based largely on ideas stemming from a high profile prototype, rather than good research evidence. But their time had come and by 2003, as our study commenced, strong political and organisational forces were spearheading their rapid diffusion in the NHS as an attempt to reduce waiting times and waiting lists for common elective procedures and to foster new forms of patient-centred care. This was all part of a much wider government drive to modernise the organisation and delivery of NHS services, which meant that NHS TCs were launched into the complex milieu of sweeping changes. Some of those changes were always bound to impact on the fledgling TCs (see Chapter Four); they included the encouragement of independent sector TCs, by such measures as the introduction of the 'G-Supp' as part of a wider governmental push towards involvement of the private sector; Payment by Results as part of stimulating improvements in organisational performance; and Patient Choice and 'Choose and Book' as part of the desire to empower patients. As a result, the story of TCs was not about a single innovation and its impact on services, but about organisational responses to a maelstrom of modernisation. Nevertheless, the dedicated extra funding and the advice from sources such as the Modernisation Agency's 'learning events' gave an opportunity for local developments that, although often very different from the Department of Health's ideal, reflected many of its intended principles. The Department might not always have things its own way but the TC programme did stimulate local change that might otherwise not have occurred.

The eight sample sites that we studied differed greatly from each other in their management styles, aspirations and pressures. Their relationships with their external milieu – the host hospital, the PCT, the SHA and neighbouring trusts – and with their own staff also varied from harmonious and constructive partnerships through to downright hostility and conflict. However, the unifying factor was that some core local 'champions' with a 'can do' mentality both within and outwith the host trust thought that the service needed to change. Once afforded the generally favourable policy environment they took up the challenge for reasons that were often rooted in local history and context (such as the pressure to find new capacity to treat patients on their own or other hospitals' waiting lists, a stalled plan to relocate surgical services or open a day surgery unit, the need to find a use for an under-used hospital building and the chance to engineer changes in local professional influence). Such motivating factors were unique to each site, but some common features emerged.

First, there were always 'contests of meaning' among the people involved, so that the emergent TC was inevitably the result of multiple, often complex, negotiations. In applying for the TC funding key players, who were themselves subject to pressures from the internal and external milieus of their organisations, inevitably needed to resolve their often conflicting views about what a TC actually meant. We noted four types: idealists who spotted a chance to improve patient care, sceptics who disagreed with TCs (another fad to be avoided, perhaps), opportunists who wanted to secure the funding to develop something (perhaps only loosely related) that they had wanted anyway and pragmatists who wanted to do whatever seemed most likely to improve services with minimum fuss. Even where there was consensus among those with the power to make the final decision, there were always tensions between their underlying motivations, rationales and intended outcomes. As a result, continually evolving and constantly negotiated clusters of decisions gradually emerged as something approaching at least some of the initial visions of a TC as seen by different levels of the health service.

Second, at each site there were always varying combinations of motives to improve quality, quantity and/or kudos. Improving quality sometimes meant 'patient-focused' approaches to care or 'modernising' patient processes, often involving the fundamental reform of traditional clinical practices and transformations in skill mix and even professional identity. Improving quantity was about increasing capacity, throughput and activity, which was usually tightly coupled to centrally driven performance management. Improving kudos for the organisation (or individuals within it) was about being more competitive (or at least not falling behind the likely competition), perhaps via their ties with external stakeholders in the local health economy or NHS hierarchy.

Third, there was always a mismatch between intent and reality. Imprecise planning, financial setbacks and widespread overcapacity meant that all eight TCs saw some of the original motivators for change, such as nurse-led care or other shifts in professional roles, evaporate. For a variety of reasons, almost none of the TCs was able to plan and predict with any consistency or precision even such basic parameters as the numbers and types of patients they would treat. Once opened, the way that the TC fared depended partly on shifts in the local health economy and the deluge of central initiatives and variable local responses (such as the financial incentives – or disincentives – for local trusts to send them patients). The outcome depended on how the managers of the TCs were able to respond to this erratic environment, which in turn largely depended on the relationships (for example, competitive or collaborative, open or secretive) they had fashioned with key local stakeholders. In this respect managers' responses to their environment were in turn shaping ('enacting') the environment with which they subsequently had to cope (Weick, 2001).

Despite the turmoil, however, TCs often saw increased throughput of patients and a decrease in waiting lists. There were some significant improvements too in the quality of the care that patients received, including well-honed individual care pathways with key milestones (albeit sometimes based controversially on US models), a nurse-led clinical pathway about which patients were fully informed before arriving at hospital, considerable redesign of the workforce and the physical environment in order to accomplish new ways of working, structured pre-operative assessment by nurses, case managers in charge of discharge planning and primary care or community trusts providing planned intermediate care. Often, however, the eventual changes were relatively superficial, failing to achieve the intended root and branch transformations. Moreover (see Table 2.1 and Chapter Five), by the end of our three-year study, most of the sites had not achieved the distinct organisational status that they had set out to achieve. In the remainder of this chapter we set out some of the theoretical conclusions one can draw from these stories in the light of existing literature on innovations in complex organisations.

The 'innovation journey'

The 'innovation journey', described by the classic Minnesota Innovation Research Programme, is an important piece of work that helps to make sense of what happened in our case studies (Van de Ven et al, 1999). Following the paths of 14 different innovations over 17 years in a variety of organisations mostly in the commercial sector, Andrew Van de Ven and colleagues observed that innovations never developed linearly but always took unexpected twists and turns in a complicated and at first sight unpredictable journey from their inception to their final uptake (or not). Hoping to find a 'non-linear dynamic system', they explored whether this might be more than just random, looking for the components in both the innovation and its environment that might help predict, and therefore perhaps control, those twists and turns. They found that an innovation is not a stable entity, nor is there a consensus about its technical potential that carries it through clear stages of development, testing, adoption and diffusion. Instead, what emerged was a very different picture, one that resonates with our own findings:

> As the developmental processes unfolded, we saw innovation ideas proliferate into many ideas. There was not only invention but reinvention; some ideas were discarded as others were reborn. Many people were involved, but most only partially: they were distracted by busy schedules as they performed other unrelated roles. The network of stakeholders involved in transactions was constantly revised. This "fuzzy set" epitomises the general environment for the innovation as multiple environments are "enacted" (Weick 1979) by various parties to the innovation. Rather than a simple, unitary, and progressive path, we recorded multiple tracks and spin-offs, some that were related and co-ordinated and others that were not.... The discrete identity of the innovation became blurred as the new and the old were integrated. (Van de Ven et al, 1999, pp 8-9)

The 'innovation journey', as Van de Ven and colleagues depict it, has a number of components that, while not usually happening in an orderly sequence, take an innovation from an initiation period through a development period, to implementation or termination (see Figure 7.1). The TCs' journeys fitted that pattern. The formulation of the national TC programme and its funding allocation (see Chapter One) was part of the *gestation* element of Van de Ven et al's initiation period, but there was local gestation too, in which aspirations to change services had already been growing and were awaiting fulfilment (see Chapter Two). The Minnesota Study found that the initiation period also requires a '*shock*', the stimulus that catalyses the innovation. For the TCs it was the sudden availability of new capital funds from the TC programme coupled usually with critical events precipitating the need to rebuild or revamp the organisation (such as increased competition, failure to meet local waiting time targets, extreme financial deficit in host organisations, or other crises for the trust) that kick-started the innovation journeys that were to transform the rumbling local and national concerns into actual TCs.

Figure 7.1 The innovation journey

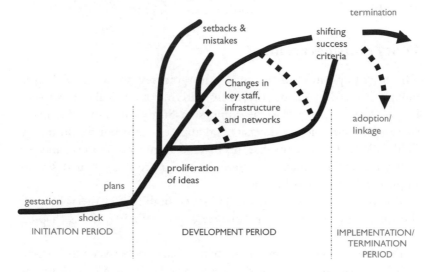

Source: Adapted from Van de Ven (1990, p 25)

The start of an innovation journey then involves local *plans,* which often consisted of business plans hastily pulled together to satisfy local and national decision makers, not necessarily to act as workable blueprints but more – as the authors of the Minnesota Study put it – to act as 'sales vehicles' aimed at 'resource controllers' (Van de Ven et al, 1999, p 23). Among the TCs such plans – and again this was consistent with the model of the innovation journey – were constantly forced to adapt in reaction to national and local policy shifts. This allowed the innovation to move to its next phase of its journey, the 'development period' characterised by the '*proliferation*' of varying ideas and activities (which epitomises the diversity that we found both within and between TCs), *setbacks* and mistakes (like the miscalculations of throughput), *shifts in the success criteria* (like the sudden requirement to admit private patients or the changes in financial arrangements wrought by Payment by Results or G-Supp), *changes in key personnel and external organisations* (most of our TCs had a rapid turnover of critical internal and external players) and the creation of a *trans-organisational community infrastructure* of innovators (such as NHS Elect).

The innovation journey ends with an implementation or termination period wherein the innovation *links the old with the new* (for example, the way that nearly all of the TCs were reabsorbed into their host trusts) and is *reinvented* to fit the local situation (a main theme of our findings). The journey ends with what Van de Ven and colleagues call the '*termination*' as the innovation either becomes mainstream or − as at St Urban's or, later, Ruckworth − ceases to exist.

Policy considerations

This brief exposition of the 'innovation journey' shows how, despite having been derived mainly from studying technical innovations in the commercial sector, the Minnesota Study's model helps make sense of the complexity, diversity and apparent disorder found in our fieldwork. It would seem that this may be a universal pattern, and yet policy makers and managers continue to ignore it in their desire to implement uniform solutions.

Moreover, we found that the TC story highlighted the following specific policy-related features that we explore further in this chapter:

* the general policy environment, which can vary between the target-led environment and the rhetoric of local initiative (top down or bottom up?);
* the implications of the way that TCs meant different things to different parts of the NHS (differing 'frames'; see Pope et al, 2006);
* the possible place of 'design principles', as opposed to design rules, in the innovation process;
* the place of rigorous mathematical modelling in NHS planning;
* the nature of planning and decision making in a volatile environment.

Top down or bottom up?

There has long been a tension in the NHS between 'top-down' approaches characterised by target setting, performance management and hierarchical line management and the 'bottom-up' model based on competition between providers and upward pressures from front-line initiatives and patient choice (Greener, 2004).[1] Figure 7.2 illustrates how these approaches sit at opposite ends of a continuum of contrasting traditions about what innovation is and how it spreads. The government's original rationale for TCs was top-down and target-led ('make it happen'), with TCs seen as vital to bringing waiting times for an elective admissions to under three months. By 2007, however, as our research was ending, the Department had espoused a shift from 'targets-driven' to 'incentives-driven' change (DH, 2006b), although whether that shift was felt as a liberating force at the local level is another question (Hoque et al, 2004). Meanwhile, the Modernisation Agency had always combined both approaches by promulgating the central government's ambition to increase productivity and reduce waiting lists while encouraging local innovation ('help it happen') by supporting front-line staff and in the stylised language of NHS modernisation ('redesign', 'radical', 'empowerment', 'innovative', 'new ways of working' and so on) to think and act differently. How NHS TCs sought to juggle and balance these different pressures became an integral part of their stories.

Based on Figure 7.2, the top-down approach ('make it happen') would sit at the linear, rationalist end of the continuum, in which 'an innovation is a more or less fixed entity, adoption is an '"event" and implementation is a rational, controllable process that is amenable to advance planning and monitoring against targets' (Greenhalgh et al, 2005, p 81). The other end of the spectrum ('let it happen') is where 'innovation, adoption, implementation and sustainability are complex, context-dependent and creative social processes that cannot be planned in detail and are not amenable to external control or manageability' (Greenhalgh et al, 2005, p 81). 'Help it happen' is a more nuanced negotiated approach that lies between these extremes. The introduction of TCs was somewhere between the 'make it happen' and the 'help it happen' models. But TCs evolved as an organisational innovation just at the time when there was an ostensible attempt to move healthcare policy towards the 'let it happen' end of the continuum (DH, 2006b). Some of the confusion and uncertainty in our case study sites seems to reflect the inherent tensions between these different approaches.

Differing 'frames'

The tension between 'make *it* happen' and 'let *it* happen' relies on the rather important question of what the '*it*' actually is. We found major differences between the concept of a TC as envisaged by the various key professions at different levels in the NHS, and between the groups we have called idealists, opportunists, pragmatists and sceptics. It is helpful to see these differences using 'frame analysis' (Goffman, 1974; Snow et al, 1986), which provides a method for exploring the interconnections and interdependencies of the differing ways that people at different levels in the health system viewed and enacted TCs, for example, the ways that macro-policy level actors, mediated by meso-level and micro-level actors, framed the problem (House et al, 1995). We have chosen one frame of particular interest at each of these three levels: the Department's government (macro) frame, the Modernisation Agency's modernising (meso) frame and trusts' local (micro) frame (Pope et al, 2006). The government frame provided the definitional components such as separating emergency and elective services, delivering faster services with increased throughput and encouraging the use of both private sector and NHS facilities. Its rationale was to reduce waiting times and create new ways of delivering care. The Modernisation Agency's frame was more focused than the government frame. It set out, for example, to list the core characteristics of a TC, but on closer inspection, these were not only vague (for example, never defining the key notion of 'high volume' activity) but also shifted subtly over time. This fuzziness allowed the many local frames to create and recreate different meanings that solved local organisational problems, and which were therefore often quite specific and quite different not only from each other but also from the macro and meso frames.

Figure 7.2: Different conceptual and theoretical bases for the spread of innovation in service organisations

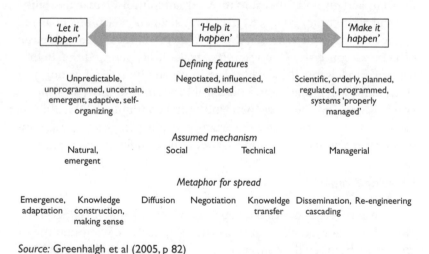

Source: Greenhalgh et al (2005, p 82)

These frames are just three of a potentially long list of existing or potential framings of TCs at all levels (such as government ministry versus Department of Health; NHS Elect versus independent sector

TCs; pragmatists versus sceptics). They shared some elements such as the separation of elective and emergency care, but the overlap was remarkably small. The Department's macro frame originated from the responsibility to execute ministerial policy and provide advice as part of the large-scale political programme of public sector reform directed by the Labour government since 1997. As such, it encompassed a number of other key health service initiatives (such as Patient Choice and the independent sector TC programme); within that frame, therefore, it made good sense to see the TCs as part of that package of initiatives. In contrast, the micro-level frame of the local TCs encompassed a quite different set of concepts and activities, shaped by the milieus and the motivators described in Chapters Two and Three, such as redevelopment of local day surgery, competitive advantage, income generation or an alteration of patient booking methods. Within this micro frame the plethora of the Department's initiatives made very little rational sense; it was just a flurry of 'must dos' with little of the consistency that was apparent to the political and civil service originators of those policies. The Modernisation Agency's meso frame, while sharing some of the aspects of both macro and micro (such as Patient Choice, new booking practices), also differed from them by having less of an emphasis on other concerns that preoccupied the TCs, such as private provision or local income generation. Rather, it focused on streamlining services, improving the patient pathways and re-engineering professional roles, sharing and disseminating best practice, and so on. Thus each frame had its own (often implicit, unspoken) definition, rationale, image, identity and terminology, and above all its own interpretation of the meanings of TCs along with their associated values, policies and activities. This is also true of the many other frames such as the PCTs, SHAs and regions, 'tribal' groups such as managers and doctors, or idealists and opportunists.

The crucial point about frames is that they both define and are defined by the sorts of concerns outlined in the preceding paragraph. Contests or negotiations of meaning between the frames helped to shape but were also shaped by the conflicting interests and forces that were pulling in differing directions. The resultants of those forces depended not only on their direction but also on the political and organisational weight that their protagonists could bring to bear. This, of course, is closely related not only to the power relations within the TC and its host trust, for example, between idealist nurses, pragmatic managers or sceptic surgeons, but also as to whether the power lay mainly at the centre (macro, top down) or with local innovators (micro, bottom up), and as we have suggested, that power base was shifting according to a series of often contradictory policy changes. But as central and local players tussled over the innovation, making or letting 'it' happen or perhaps preventing 'it' from happening, they each perceived a different 'it' from within their various frames.

Figure 7.3: Three frames with examples of their varied needs from the TC programme

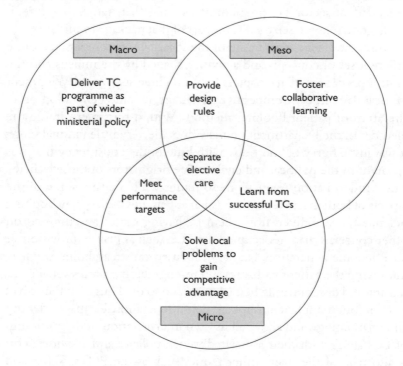

The pendulum has continued to swing between declarations of clear central policy direction and devolving initiative to the NHS front line (Darzi, 2008). By the end of our study in 2006 the Department had already begun to swing back towards local empowerment and 'local innovation' (DH, 2005b). What difference might this make to the way organisational innovations such as TCs develop? The first thing to note is that despite their birth during a top-down phase of policy making, there always was considerable variation between TCs locally, and between what the centre expected and what the TCs were prepared to give them (Pope et al, 2006). This suggests to us that, if the NHS TCs are anything to go by, the Department had little choice but to retreat from a 'make it happen' model that had already lost much of its directive power.[2] *De facto*, and some would say perversely, our

TCs displayed most of the features of the new more devolved model even before it was introduced, a case perhaps of policy following (and legitimising) practice rather than leading it. It is worth noting that Ferlie et al (2006, p 71), in their study of seven healthcare providers engaged with London Choice, found, as we did, that 'some of the DTC capacity was pre-existing and relabelled for "Choice"'.

TCs were given a clear policy objective (for example, the reduction of waiting times), a set of principles related to their development (the Modernisation Agency's *desiderata*, see Appendix 1) and a timeline to do it in. Yet they all evolved differently from national blueprint to local product (some rapidly, some slowly, some never) to suit diverse local needs and agendas, and striving to stand out as much as to conform. This is nothing new. Pressman and Wildavsky's (1984) classic study of policy implementation showed how the efforts of the US federal government's Economic Development Administration to create jobs for the long-term unemployed in Oakland suffered setbacks that were not only costly but typical of the problems encountered in federal–local projects, equivalent to Department of Health–local trust projects.[3] Warren (1974) suggests that the most important maxim to be learned from their tale of programme failure is that:

> ... implementation should not be divorced from policy.... In other words, programs fail too frequently because too much respect, effort and enthusiasm are given to program design, obtaining initial support from the participating community and funding, while the implementation stage is regarded as the easy part involving only routine, technical questions that can always be worked out later as long as the program itself is sound. (Warren, 1974, p 1090)

While not all our TCs 'failed', Warren's view resonates strongly with our findings. Moreover, the hiatus between top-down policy and local product was not helped by the dissolution of the Modernisation Agency and its TC team midstream, nor by the unclear role of the SHAs. Both tended to remove whatever weak meso-level connectors had existed. Brooks and Bate's (1994) analysis of a change programme in the British civil service found a similar picture. They suggested that the British civil service was unlikely to move towards transformation (planned or unplanned), but that it would either stay the same or take on less radical elements of the change programme. Exworthy et al's (2002) study of the adoption of UK policies to address health inequalities shows a remarkably similar pattern. Despite national policies to reduce health inequalities being treated as a centrally driven innovation and despite strong alignment in the values underpinning both central and local policy making on inequalities, there was little or none of the intended direct vertical cascade of the programme. In reality, what central government saw as uptake of the innovative policies to reduce inequalities was actually a rebranding of existing initiatives to fit the new category (and budgets) assigned to 'inequalities initiatives'. It seems that wherever one looks, *plus ça change, plus c'est la même chose....*

Such disconnections between central policy and implementation raise big questions about the role of the centre, which – at least in the area of innovation – appears not only to lack directive power but also to have relatively weak influence on what happens locally. The implication must be that the centre should concentrate on outlining and facilitating implementation (setting boundaries and common rules and frameworks) rather than trying to directly determine it.

That being said, we cannot simply dismiss national policy as always irrelevant or unhelpful. For instance, the systematic review of the diffusion of innovations in health service organisations by Greenhalgh et al (2004, 2005, p 14) reported on several empirical studies that measured the effect of the policy context on the adoption of a particular innovation. They found that:

> ... a policy "push" occurring at the early stage of implementation of an innovation initiative can increase its chances of success, perhaps most crucially by making a dedicated funding stream available. External mandates (political "must-dos") increase the predisposition, but not the capacity, of an organisation to adopt an innovation; such mandates (or the fear of them) may divert activity away from innovations as organisations seek to second-guess what they will be required to do next rather than focus on locally generated ideas and priorities. (Greenhalgh et al, 2004, p 610)

This applied also to TCs: the centre of the NHS may not have achieved quite what it had planned, but it *did* make a difference. Not only was there significant capital funding that enabled the TCs to be built or refurbished, but also other kinds of significant resources were made available to help them develop, such as the Modernisation Agency programme, NHS Elect and the AmbiCentres International initiative.[4] It could be argued, therefore, that the centre did quite a lot to 'help it happen', but was thwarted by the myriad other initiatives that made it almost impossible for TCs to happen as anyone had originally envisaged. In such circumstances, it was perhaps inevitable that local solutions would emerge that moved towards the initial ideal of a TC but also tried to meet the many other ideals that were sometimes not just pulling in different – indeed contrary – directions, but creating potential local catastrophes.

Decreed design rules or shared design principles?

The processes and outcomes of innovation depend on how an organisation deals with what has been called the coordination–autonomy dilemma (Puranam et al, 2006). How might the NHS deal with the competing need for coordination mechanisms such as standard operating procedures, rules, routines and targets, and still accept the need for the autonomy that allows people to try new things and develop mutual learning and a shared (rather than imposed) language? Any national policy guidance 'can only set the parameters within which local organisations will work' (DH, 2006b, p 3) and perhaps, therefore, a new and more constructive way of conceiving the task might be in the form of 'design principles' for innovation that forgo directives in favour of imperatives distilled from experience and practice. Design principles enable one to say: 'If you want to achieve innovation Y in situation S, something like X might help' (Bate and Robert, 2007; Bevan et al, 2007; Plsek et al, 2007). They move away from behavioural rules and a mindset of control (which many perceive in negative terms) towards an emphasis on sharing knowledge about what has worked, and more importantly, why, and how it has worked in the way that it has. Such an approach, which is a more positive approach to organisational learning,[5] pushes all stakeholders to ask:

- Are there design principles for implementing this kind of organisational innovation? If so what are they?
- What key considerations should be borne in mind?
- What are the tried and tested design exemplars (for something like this innovation) that we already know about?

Answers to such questions are most likely to come from those who have close experience of managing the innovation in question, which suggests that communities of practice may have a great deal to offer. Communities of practice have been described as:

> ... groups of people who share a concern, a set of problems, or a passion about a topic, and who deepen their understanding and knowledge of this area by interacting.... These people don't necessarily work together on a day-to-day basis, but they get together because they find value in their interactions. As they spend time together, they typically share information, insight, and advice. They solve problems. They help each other. They discuss their situation, their aspirations, their needs. They think about common issues. They explore ideas and act as sounding boards to each other. They may create tools, standards, generic designs, manuals, and other documents; or they may just keep what they know as a tacit understanding they share. (Wenger et al, 2002, pp 4/5)

They enable practitioners to develop and share tacit as well as explicit knowledge and practices that can contribute substantially to organisational learning and development in health services (le May, 2009). There was some evidence of such learning within some of the TCs, but more proactive promotion of communities of practice across different sites may have helped avert some of the problems or deal with them more effectively. It might be argued that the Modernisation Agency, and in particular their 'learning events', were intended to work with managers to seek out and share the answers to questions about what had worked for TCs. But we did not see this happen. The process that they used was not able to get to the heart of 'why' and 'how' the design principles for TCs and why they were succeeding or not. At the learning events, for example, where it might have been possible to encourage managers to reflect together and share details of how and why some design principles worked or not, and to develop them collectively, there was reluctance to do so. This was no community of practice. The events were carefully stage managed and if there was a sharing of the deeper concerns or the why and how of developing TCs, it happened mainly in the relatively short periods of informal networking, and not as part of the explicit sharing of practice. Perhaps in a performance-driven, competitive NHS, the organisers and the participants were careful not to delve too deeply for fear of disturbing the illusion of a shining innovation and letting the side down. Instead, the public processes seemed to us to collude in keeping up appearances rather than genuinely striving to develop realistic design principles. While the learning events tended to focus on positive exemplars, in contrast at other (mainly internal) fora we heard chief executives and senior clinical managers ranting about their adverse environment and its dire effects on their TC – on one memorable occasion even using graphic images from the film *The Perfect Storm* to describe the policy context.

Neither the centre nor its meso-level agents such as the Modernisation Agency or the SHAs (DH, 2006b, p 3) were – for whatever reason – able to foster the collective development of design principles. Arguably, and despite the powerful unitary intentions of the centre, this inability had a divisive effect that increased the autonomy at the local level. It led to fragmentation and loss of some of the gains that might have been made as the result of the stakeholders in the local health economies working more closely together on specific issues such as TC development. This may seem surprising to some observers who claim that the Department has been too 'hands on'. But our observations of the development of TCs suggests that, paradoxically, it was the very plethora of central directives lacking in common design principles that made it possible (and essential) for each locality to steer its own apparently autonomous course – whatever course seemed to local managers most likely to optimise the achievement of their particular confluence of conflicting demands.

If the NHS hierarchy were instead to encourage the development of design principles, it could avoid too great an emphasis on benchmarking and prescriptive detail of the sort that often caused the TCs to abreact. It could also – as the Modernisation Agency was so often unable to do – reconcile the twin pulls of, on the one hand, advice, guidelines and support and, on the other, targets and performance management. An example of a practical application of this design principles approach (Bevan et al, 2007) was a national project whose goal was to create an improvement 'product' (the 'ten high impact changes') that would have particular appeal to chief executives and senior leaders of NHS trusts, thereby helping to (a) close the gap between strategic intentions and isolated front-line initiatives, and (b) create better, quicker, more sustainable change. The design process entailed formulating high-level universal principles that could be tailored and adapted to a wide variety of local contexts by those directly involved in their implementation. Although the centre, for example, through the Modernisation Agency, brought value in providing the broad design principles, it was left to front-line practitioners to implement changes as they saw fit and in ways that they decided. This allowed local ownership and choice that encouraged the various levels of the large and highly pluralistic system that is the NHS to work in a reasonably coordinated yet self-managing and semi-autonomous manner.

Mathematical modelling in NHS planning

While we do not discuss it here, part of our study of TCs used operational research methods including probability theory, mathematical modelling and thought experiments to describe the flows of patients through their treatment pathways, and to predict how variations in factors such as length of stay, number of 'beds', variability in the scheduling of admissions and heterogeneous case mix would impact on the way TCs functioned (Utley and Gallivan, 2004; Gallivan, 2005; Gallivan and Utley, 2005; Utley et al, 2005, 2008, 2009). This showed not only that it is possible mathematically to model optimised patient flows and bed capacity (see Box 7.1), but that there were some circumstances under which the introduction of a TC might be predicted to offer little if any benefit to the local health economy and could create serious problems of over-capacity. Indeed this did occur in just the kinds of sites that the model predicted. Yet the planning capacity of NHS management in the frenetic environment in which TCs were being developed meant that policy makers and managers could not appreciate the usefulness or relevance of this kind of modelling, despite its apparent logical strength. The local political and clinical context, motivations and environments made it impossible for operations researchers to carry any weight in the complex evolution of plans, negotiations and implementation.

It is interesting to draw a comparison between healthcare and transport planning, another area concerned with providing a large-scale and complex public service. Before the introduction of any major change in a transport system, huge amounts of high quality mathematical modelling and operational research and planning are carried out. Major research centres, such as the Transport Research Laboratory, have been established, employing hundreds of scientists whose work focuses on the topic of transport, and there are many more working in local authorities and the private sector. In contrast, there are relatively few centres in the healthcare sector able to carry out relevant mathematical modelling. Such centres as there are mostly rely on consultancy funding, which is rarely forthcoming since operations research can often highlight potential problem areas that make the results unwelcome, and not just for TCs.[6] Although such work can help avoid pitfalls and promote effective policy, a dispassionate critical review of proposed changes can be highly challenging, particularly if – for all the kinds of reasons that we found for the TCs – an organisation has already convinced itself the innovation's merits. One of the key roles of such analysis is to discard options that show unforeseen and detrimental effects on a system's predicted performance. The ethos of this kind of work is that while an idea that works in theory may possibly not work in practice, we can be sure that an idea that doesn't even work in theory has very little chance in practice. If the enthusiasm and planning for TCs had been informed by such independent analysis it is conceivable that some of the eventual problems could have been avoided. The detrimental policy clash between the TC and choice programmes, so easily predictable in 2002 and so clearly manifest by 2006, is stark

Box 7.1: An example of operational research modelling applied to TCs

The accompanying figure shows mathematically that, all other things being equal, if there is one single centre rather than two, then fewer beds are needed for a given population of heterogeneous patients; in other words, there are economies of scale. Hence, one argument against the introduction of a TC alongside a hospital (or, perhaps against opening more than one TC to serve the same population, as happened in large cities and also when Robbleswade, Northendon and other TCs were serving overlapping geographical areas) is that having separate pools of capacity for different groups of patient might well require a *greater* number of beds overall to cope with the inevitable variation among patients. However, it can also be shown that if, by introducing a TC, one selects more homogeneous groups of patients (so that, for example, if one can predict exactly how long each patient will stay), then one can use *fewer* beds. Such complex contradictory effects can be modelled to inform the size of a TC for a given population, but such planning aids were not taken into consideration at any of our case study TCs.

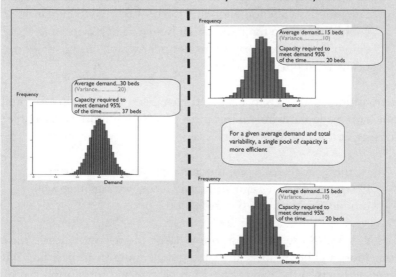

evidence that operational research could have a significant role to play but is under-used in the UK health service. However, as the next section will suggest, there are many reasons besides a reluctance to risk hearing unwelcome forecasts, why such rational analyses are ignored.

Planning and decision making in a volatile environment

Few would challenge the contention that better, more rigorous, more intelligent, more systematic planning over a less compressed time period, with more stakeholder engagement and relationship building, would have reduced the gap between plan and reality, and averted many of the TCs' ensuing problems. However, it still leaves a question as to how far the TCs could ever, for example, have accurately predicted, and subsequently managed, their workload and activity levels when their external milieu was subject to so many unanticipated changes. "More and better planning" is therefore only part of the solution; the other part is how those involved can get better at managing innovation and change in conditions of high uncertainty and growing volatility and complexity.

One key point centres on whether the NHS can plan future innovations better. As one respected observer, José Fonseca, has noted:

> Regardless of whether innovation is thought of as a "hard" scientific and technological process, a rational management process, or a "soft" intuitive human process, all these perspectives have in common the assumption that innovation is a phenomenon that can be subjected to human control. It is taken for granted that humans can purposefully design, in advance, the conditions under which change will occur. (Fonseca, 2002, p 3)

Even assuming the TCs' plans could have been more accurate, could they have made the whole innovation process any more controllable? Fonseca, at least, would say not:

> ... these processes ... are fundamentally uncertain, making it impossible to design in advance the settings that will produce innovations. (Fonseca, 2002, p 9)

The TCs and those in a position to assist them could clearly have done more and better local and strategic planning than they did,[7] but there are limits to the extent to which change and innovation can be planned with any reasonable degree of accuracy. All of our case study sites got their numbers wrong, sometimes very wrong. Better marketing and business analysis would undoubtedly have made a difference, and those involved acknowledged this, but the problems do seem to run deeper than being a simple case of poor planning and bad management. Perhaps this is in the nature of complex processes, where no amount of planning and data gathering could have accurately predicted the numbers.[8] As Richard Beckhard put it:

> I have learned through experience and the experiences of those I have consulted and taught that the correlation between a good plan and a good outcome is, to say the least, unreliable. This helped me to understand … why so many organisations' strategic plans don't end up in effective actions. (Beckhard, 1997, pp 143-4)

Beckhard's point is that getting the numbers wrong is not about bad planning or woolly thinking (although as our TCs show, it can at least partly be so) but in the complex, unpredictable nature of innovation and change processes themselves, which cannot be ignored in the hope that they become simpler and more predictable. Instead the unpredictability must be proactively managed – as was indeed instinctively recognised by many of the TC managers as they strove to allow their TCs to evolve and survive in the changing environment.

Rosabeth Moss Kanter and colleagues wrote in similar vein:

> While the literature often portrays an organisation's quest for change like a brisk march along a well-marked path, those in the middle of change are more likely to describe their journey as a laborious crawl towards an elusive, flickering goal, with many wrong turns and missed opportunities along the way. Only rarely does an organisation know exactly where it's going, or how it should get there…. Those external, uncontrollable, and powerful forces are not to be underestimated, and they are one reason why some researchers have questioned the manageability of change at all. (Kanter et al, 1992, pp 373-4).[9]

External forces played their part in the TC planning debacle, but internal managers must also bear some of the responsibility for the inflation of activity forecasts and the increasingly optimistic plans they produced to please resource controllers. Those making the case for TCs had to satisfy a tense web of forces pulling in various directions: the interests and concerns of key players in the internal and external milieus, the often mutually contradictory motivations of the centre and the host organisations and the subsequent policy shifts and performance management, all tended to lead to over-optimistic forecasts of benefits that included the unrealistic throughput figures. Clearly, the story of TCs is not just about planning or the lack of it, but about innovation politics and complex processes of dispute, negotiation and contest.

Taking these factors into account, Table 7.1 summarises two contrasting perspectives on the management of innovation: the *planning view* and the *complex systems view*. The complex systems view

Table 7.1: Two contrasting perspectives on managing organisational innovation

	Planning	Complex systems
Assumptions about the task	Rational, ordered, controllable, predictable, linear and sequential, and therefore manageable	Disordered and messy, unforeseeable, unplannable, uncontrollable, flexible and emergent, and therefore barely manageable
Approach	Programmatic, rule-centred; building robust project management systems	Pragmatic, human-centred, building 'supportive social arrangements' (Kanter, 1988)
Key focus	Structure, system and rules	Process and affiliation
Effectiveness	Better planning, tighter control and accountability	Better preparation, intense network interaction, communication and relationship building
Key skills	Project management and organisational skills	Political and networking skills
Sees itself as	Professional and well-organised	Entrepreneurial and opportunistic
Sees the other as	Sloppy	Dogmatic

of the planning and decision-making processes for TCs is a long way from the traditional model that has its roots in the classical rational economic theory of the firm with its broad set of assumptions that goals, alternatives, risk, order of preference and data are generally known and clear. It is also quite distant from the bounded rationality model which assumes decision makers have limitations that constrain rationality and therefore may not consider all possible alternatives, settling instead for a satisfactory not optimal solution. Like Lindblom's description of what he calls 'the science of muddling through' (Lindblom, 1959), in which decision makers make do with solutions that are sufficiently satisfactory (that is, that 'satisfice'), bounded rationality allows for open and dynamic planning, with decision makers changing direction as new information and intelligence flow in, all of which flexibility is still more rational than the complex systems model. The TCs displayed some elements of the rational and bounded rationality models. But what we found had more in common with sense making and decision making in situations of high uncertainty, ambiguity and volatility (Weick, 2001), where detailed planning-based models of organisational change and innovation can be unnecessarily burdensome, unreliable or plain useless.[10]

The story of the NHS TCs is therefore strongly reminiscent of the 'irrational' (Brunsson, 1982; Bryman, 1984), and 'garbage can' models of organised anarchy, organic innovation and decision processes first described in the organisation studies literature of the 1970s and 1980s (for example, Cohen et al, 1972). The 'garbage can model' was developed to explain patterns of decision making and innovation where goals, problems, alternatives and solutions are ill defined and each step of a decision or organisation change is ambiguous; where there is unclear, poorly understood technology; where cause–effect relationships within the organisation are difficult to identify; where an explicit data base that applies to decisions is not available; and where not only are staff too busy to allocate more than a limited time to any one problem or task, but where staff changeovers mean that their participation in any given decision will be fluid and limited. We believe that local managers involved in the NHS TC programme would recognise the garbage can model since most of these conditions clearly applied for most of the time we studied them.

> The contents of a real garbage can consist of whatever people have tossed into the can. A decision-making garbage can is much the same. The four streams – choices, problems, participants and solutions – flow toward the garbage can. Whatever is in the can when a decision is needed

contributes to that decision. The garbage can model sees decision making in organisations as chaotic: solutions look for problems to solve, and decision makers make choices based on the arbitrary mix of the four streams in the can (Champoux, 1996, pp 403-4).

The original model centred on organisational decision making, but provides a neat explanation for the looseness, randomness and disconnection that characterised what happened to the TCs as streams of problems, potential solutions, participants and choice opportunities happen to coincide (or not):

> Thus when viewing the organisation as a whole and considering its high level of uncertainty, one sees problems arise that are not solved and solutions tried that do not work. Organisation decisions are disorderly and not the result of a logical step-by-step sequence. Events may be so ill defined and complex that decisions, problems, and solutions act as independent events. When they connect, some problems are solved, but many are not. (Daft, 1995, p 381)

This was particularly evident in the almost serendipitous confluence of local factors that led to the decisions to open the TCs. One can point easily to the streams of problems (the need to be competitive, to improve throughput, to refurbish a building, to tame the orthopaedic surgeons), choices (a new ward? a larger day surgery unit? a change in out-patients? a TC? a new deal with the independent sector?), solutions (acquire new funds to build a TC? send elective patients elsewhere? import foreign surgical teams? introduce nurse practitioners?) and participants (a sceptical chief executive replaced by an idealist, a nearby trust deciding to send and then not to send patients, an SHA being able – or not – to direct patient flows towards the TC).

However, the picture was not just of serendipitous mixing of the contents of the 'garbage can'. There was also a large measure of continual intelligent sense making and skilful decision making to steer the innovation forward on whatever seemed the best available course. We need therefore to consider not only how people arrive at decisions or make plans, but also the follow-on question of how people might manage an organisational innovation amid a random mix of influences, and where they lack the power or capacity to analyse, prioritise and make rational choices via an explicit path. Behavioural theories have portrayed organisational actors as puppets on a string, helpless playthings of social forces, corks bobbing on a mighty sea – coping, trying to keep their heads above water, surviving rather than managing (Marsh, 2006). Yet we found very little evidence of this even among NHS managers dealing with an organisational innovation amid unpredictable and uncontrollable events where normal rational planning assumptions and disciplines did not apply. Rather, our impression was of some quite artful skippering of a vessel tossed about by the ever-changing winds and currents. Many (at least those who didn't fall overboard) coped well, and many (although not all) thereby helped their TCs to survive what one chief executive called 'the perfect storm' of adverse circumstances. This view of innovation to which we are pointing does not reject the description of complex, almost chaotic organisational reality, but reveals that in the face of adversity, the managers did not give up or even settle for muddling through or clinging on. In contrast to the classic view of powerlessness (Blauner, 1964), they revealed positive energy and resolve characterised by resilience, care, commitment, optimism and respect – indeed even the kind of 'transcendence' and 'positive spirals of flourishing' reminiscent of 'positive organisational scholarship' (Cameron et al, 2003, p 4; Conner, 2006). While such an approach did not always pay off, it does describe a positive side to the process that needs to be included in the emerging picture of the management of innovation processes.

Conceptualising key success factors in healthcare innovation

Drawing on the model that Greenhalgh et al (2005, p 200) developed to identify key success factors in the emergence and diffusion of organisational innovations like TCs, we can point to some wider insights into the management of organisational innovations more generally.

- As an *organisational innovation* NHS TCs had a number of key attributes that encouraged adoption, including their relative advantage (the provision of fast, reliable and efficient treatment and improved care for patients) that were compatible with the values of most NHS staff. TCs also had a number of less explicit positive attributes such as their usefulness in challenging entrenched professional roles. This general consensus may explain why – allied to a strong central directive and their high potential for reinvention locally – TCs appeared so rapidly and in greater numbers than expected. But TCs were also a relatively complex innovation requiring multi-disciplinary working as well as 'buy-in' from a wide variety of external stakeholders, and so always had the potential to stimulate resistance, especially from those who felt threatened by the changes it brought, or associated TCs with a perception that they were (by sometimes unwarranted association with the private sector) undermining some deeply held NHS values.

- *Adoption and assimilation* of innovations can be dictatorial (where individuals in organisations are told to adopt) or collective (where everyone must decide whether to adopt or not). Idealists, opportunists, pragmatists and sceptics, as well as conflicting interests around professional roles and status, reduced the likelihood of collective adoption decisions within any given site so the adoption decisions were typically relatively dictatorial, but because the perceived characteristics and meaning of TCs was so varied, it nevertheless tended to be 'complex, iterative, organic and untidy' rather than a single event (Greenhalgh et al, 2005, p 103).

- *Diffusion* of innovations that have been introduced as strategically planned formal developments (as in the case of NHS TCs via *The NHS Plan*) tends to be via vertical dissemination networks. This was true of NHS TCs but later their spread was also influenced by 'lateral' connections, particularly when NHS trusts saw TCs as an opportunity to achieve any number of local objectives and reacted accordingly.

- The *inner context* (which we here have called the internal milieu) was such that virtually all NHS TCs were introduced into large organisations with high degrees of specialisation, functional differentiation and professionalisation but typically with few slack resources and limited ability to manage a long-term organisational change process and to evaluate it over time. So while the early planning and building phases of TCs were typified by not just by clinical expertise but also by strong project management, the latter typically ebbed away as the facilities developed. Conflicting goals as well as increasing competition for management time reduced the organisations' absorptive capacity (Pressman and Wildavsky, 1984), so that system-wide implications of NHS TCs were often not thought through.

- Another aspect of the context is the *physical environment*. One of the features of the TCs was the mutual influence between the staff and their surroundings – 'space both creates *and* is created by human agency' (Halford and Leonard, 2006, p 13). People who work in 'modernised' surroundings not only tend to act differently but contribute to the way those surroundings develop. The look and feel of the building, which was part of the vision and stimulus for many of the protagonists of TCs, played an important part in symbolising and encouraging the different ways of working that TCs entailed. Examples such as huge and airy spaces, purposively constructed layouts to suit the patient pathways, and deliberately 'consumer-oriented décor' were all part of the process of change. As Pope et al (2010, p 68) have suggested, in most of the TCs '[t]he new culture became an inevitable consequence of the environment that was itself enacted by that culture' and the power of that element of the change should not be overlooked.

- The *outer context* (external milieu) was characterised by a very strong central, top-down drive that encouraged (at times insisted on or reinforced through national performance targets) the early uptake of TCs.[11] However, apparently conflicting national policies have undermined the viability of at least some TCs, especially policies that were controversial both within and outside the NHS (the expansion of private sector TCs, for example).

- Features of the *implementation*[12] *and institutionalisation* process included strong reliance on influential enthusiasts and supporters (particularly among clinicians) and significant recruitment and/or training in the early stages. Middle managers in the host trusts were sometimes not well disposed to what they saw as the freedoms and opportunities afforded to their counterparts in the TCs. However, they also saw the benefits of the innovation in helping them to meet targets such as waiting times and patient throughput, and in challenging entrenched clinicians. Although some TCs established outcomes measurement as a core activity – such as the patient satisfaction surveys that they all conducted – there was little strategic assessment of their impact on wider healthcare systems and most of their information systems could not provide the necessary data to do so.[13]

- Finally, as far as the *role of external agencies* was concerned, although significant funding was made available for capital projects, central support for addressing the challenges of implementation was mixed and piecemeal and fell away after the demise of the Modernisation Agency. And as we have shown, the meanings attached to NHS TCs by external agents such as the Modernisation Agency, the Department of Health and SHAs were often at odds with those of TC managers and staff.

Conclusions

So what does this analytic overview of TCs as an organisational innovation tell us about how to manage such advances in the future? First, that even a combination of (a) widely acknowledged high relative advantage, (b) close compatibility with the values, norms and needs of adopters and (c) a high potential to adapt, refine and modify an innovation is insufficient to guarantee its successful implementation and spread. Rather, it is the interaction between an innovation, its intended adopters and its context that determines the adoption rate and success or otherwise of its local implementation.

Second, although the early diffusion of organisational innovations can be accelerated by a strong top-down policy directive, capital funding, central facilitation and powerful local champions in the form of senior clinicians and chief executives, successful implementation requires consistent strategic and front-line change management skills. These are often in short supply in the NHS, but where external change agents are brought in to support implementation they require a common language and values system, and shared meanings.[14] This was not always true, say, of the Modernisation Agency staff who, amid all their facilitation of networking and collaboration to support adopters, often did not recognise and address the pervasive contests of meaning. Indeed they sometimes seemed to speak – or even seek to impose – a different language.

Third, although many of the typical structural characteristics of a large acute hospital with its specialisation and functional differentiation should in theory increase the likelihood of the adoption of organisational innovations, the typically limited – or absent – 'slack resources' in NHS trusts reduce the receptivity and hence the assimilation of the innovation. In other words, while there appear to be well structured groups of specialised staff, they may lack the time and skills to deal with the organisational problems that inevitably arise. This again points to the potentially important supplementary role of external networks, communities of practice and practical support.

Fourth, conflicting parallel policy initiatives and resulting uncertainty can militate against the ability of those leading implementation at the local level to respond as adaptively as they would like, especially if such initiatives are controversial and have mixed support.

Fifth, implementing complex organisational innovations that cut across pre-existing local and regional organisational boundaries requires a greater focus on connecting the relevant parts of the NHS to operate as an innovation *system* rather than as a loose collection of fragments. Such connectivity is increased in a policy environment based less on top-down directives and more design principles that can absorb, for example, patient views and local incentives. Again, this implies the need for better managed networks and communities of practice that address the different frames of meaning of the key players.

Finally, both the planning and complex system perspectives (see Table 7.1) have weaknesses and omissions, but it is in the discrepancies and differences between the two that we may find some important lessons for managing organisational innovations (Seo et al, 2004; Poole and Van de Ven, 2004). For example, the 'rational, linear planning model' of innovation is especially unsuited to 'volatile environments' (Augustine et al, 2005) that are not stable, consistent or well understood, not least when they were never designed for change but for maintaining order. Many in the NHS would argue that they are experiencing a more volatile environment than ever before, with so many structural and leadership changes, and so many unknowns. Moreover, any innovation such as TCs itself adds to this volatility. If so, the rational model will always be found wanting, no matter how skilled people are in its use.

Equally, however, the complex systems perspective is on its own unlikely to be effective, leading to missed targets, drift and growing resentment among other stakeholders about the lack of knowledge, coordination and an overall systems view. This also brings us back to our earlier point that implementation cannot be divorced from policy. Organisational innovation needs a judicious mix of the planning and the complex systems views of policy making and implementation. One needs plans and controls (more than we found in our study) but – and this is the important point – only for those things that can be planned and controlled. One also needs the processes and skills that come from the complex systems perspective (which again were not greatly in evidence in our sites), which can deal with all the emergent, unpredictable aspects of the innovation implementation process. How this judicious mix, which we might call 'agile innovation', might look in practice is the question to which we now finally turn.

Notes

[1] The notion of 'top down' is, of course, relative. To those working in a clinic, the local trust managers might be seen as top-down managers, to whom, in turn, it is the centre of the NHS that is acting in that way. We use the term here in that latter, broader, context of the relationship between central policy makers and local senior managers.

[2] At the same time this confirmed Pressman and Wildavsky's (1984, pp 126-7) witty description of the self-delusion that so often accompanies top-down policy implementation of the 'make it happen' variety: 'The view from the top is exhilarating. Divorced from the problems of implementation, federal bureau heads, leaders of international agencies and prime ministers in poor countries think great thoughts together. But they have trouble imagining the

sequence of events that will bring their paths to fruition. Other men, they believe, will tread the path once they have so brightly lit the way.'

[3] The authors suggested four possible reasons for central objectives not being realised. One explanation is the assertion of faulty implementation. Another explanation may be that aspirations were set too high. Third, the possibility of a mismatch between means and ends calls into question the adequacy of the original policy design (perhaps implementation was good but the theory on which it was based was bad). Finally, could a different set of initial conditions have achieved the predicted results?

[4] AmbiCentres International was formed in 2004 to 'carry forward our faith in the provision of healthcare through Treatment Centres'. The website (no longer available) included: (a) a database of TCs with information on services; (b) a library of information to aid best practice; and (c) a meeting place for anyone interested in TCs where information can be exchanged (www.ambicentres. net/section.cfm?id=25, last accessed September 2006).

[5] This idea of a positive – glass is half full – mindset has created a whole new area of research and practice known as 'positive organisational scholarship', which its advocates argue is a transformative mindset especially for bureaucracies such as the NHS. Certainly this approach to TC innovation would have been very different from the one that we observed, with far greater emphasis among those other than the 'idealists' on the possibilities and opportunities that TCs brought, and far less on scarcity, negative politics and constraint. See Cameron et al (2003); Bright and Cameron (2009); www.bus.umich.edu/Positive/

[6] One related piece of work for Patient Choice highlighted the difficulties that might arise, many of which came to pass. The study (Gallivan and Utley, 2002) supports the view that there was potential for a large amount of capacity to go unused. The potential difficulties identified were as follows: the possible promotion of cartel arrangements, provision of incentives to defer treatment for patients with the greatest clinical need, quality migration, 'uneconomics' of scale, chaotic queue behaviour, the potential for confusion and misunderstandings, how a 'first come first served' choice policy can restrict patient satisfaction, how choice can restrict access, capacity implications, payment for activity rather than capacity, the stability of funding mechanisms, unexpected dysfunctional system performance, choice benefiting patients only if accurate information about their options is available, the consequences of increased patient travel, conflict with other goals of the health system, HR implications and medico-legal problems. The reaction of the organisation to follow-up work on capacity requirements was to stop responding to

communications; the invoice for the work remains unpaid. From the outside, this seemed consistent with an organisation in a state of denial.

[7] If any further evidence of the deficiencies in central strategic planning were needed witness the decision in 2006 to cancel seven of the 24 planned local independent sector TCs. By 2007, the third wave of independent sector TCs had been cancelled altogether (Evans, 2007).

[8] Like the weather, top-down planning approaches always carry the possibility that the reality will not live up to the forecast. To continue the weather forecast metaphor, Quinn (1980) notes that, 'A good deal of corporate planning is like a ritual rain dance. It has no effect on the weather that follows, but those who engage in it think it does.... Moreover, much of the advice related to corporate planning is directed at improving the dancing, not the weather.'

[9] Kanter (1983, 1989) also analysed hundreds of case studies and failed to find any evidence for the success of rational planning models in most of them. Greenhalgh et al (2005, p 80) cite this work as 'some of the best empirical evidence on how innovation arises in complex systems'.

[10] Balogun and Johnson (2005) – explicitly recognising the tendency of intended strategies to lead to unintended consequences – studied the social processes of interaction between middle managers (the equivalent of many of our TC managers) as change recipients as they try to make sense of a change intervention. In common with much contemporary organisational change theory, they found that 'managing change is less about directing and controlling and more about facilitating recipient sensemaking processes' (p 1596).

[11] This is in contrast to some other innovations in healthcare; for example, integrated care pathways that initially arose peripherally and were spread informally via the professional networks of clinician enthusiasts (Greenhalgh et al, 2005, p 203).

[12] Defined as the 'early usage activities that often follow the adoption decision' (Meyers et al, 1999).

[13] This is important as research suggests that accurate and timely information (through efficient data collection and review systems) on the impact of the implementation increases the chance of successfully making it routine (Greenhalgh et al, 2005, p 15).

[14] As we have argued in this report, and as Greenhalgh et al (2005, p 9) suggest, 'if the meaning attached to the innovation by individual adopters is congruent with the meaning attached by top management, service users and other stakeholders, assimilation is more likely'. Often that congruency was missing.

EIGHT

Implications for policy, practice and research

What follows is a series of practical tips that reflect what appeared to us to have affected the outcome of the TCs' stories. If many seem just common sense, we can only point to the old saying that common sense is not always common. Some points are included because there appeared to be clear benefits when they were well executed, but many are included because the failure to deploy them at one or more sites may well have undermined the intended improvements. These general points highlight some of the important lessons for future organisational innovations in health services, but undoubtedly the most useful lessons will be those that readers will have drawn from relating their own experiences to the TC stories as they read them. It is those varied and specific experiences and contexts that will bring out the relevant lessons for readers' own organisations.

For policy makers

1 Top-down target-led central innovations will inevitably be re-crafted at the local level to suit local needs and build on existing initiatives; they need therefore to retain appropriate flexibility (headroom) if they are to be crafted while still successfully fulfilling their core objectives (see Chapters Two and Three).

2 Policy makers should try to facilitate local innovation using not blueprints and design rules but '*design principles*' that acknowledge the likelihood that rational planning of innovations will be limited in both its feasibility and its applicability in the volatile environment of health service management (see Chapter Seven).

3 Even where an organisational innovation has all the attributes of likely success (for example, that it is widely acknowledged to have high relative advantage; seems compatible with the values, norms and perceived needs of those who are expected to adopt it; and has the potential to be adapted to a range of local requirements) there is no guarantee that it will work. It is therefore also necessary to explore very carefully the potential interaction between the innovation, its intended adopters and its context when assessing the likelihood of

successful implementation. It is also vital to strive to ensure that related policies do not undermine the intended innovation (see Chapters Four and Five).

4 More careful assessments of the likely impact of new policies on policies that are already working their way through the system should be undertaken before those new policies are introduced nationally (see Chapters Four and Five).

5 There should be more rigorous evaluation of innovative policies while they are on the drawing board. Where this reveals strong evidence – for example, from modelling techniques – that problems will arise from the widespread implementation of an innovation, due caution should be diligently exercised, not swept aside (see Chapter Seven).

6 Specific training may be required among managers at all levels of the service, as successful implementation of organisation-wide innovations requires a high level of both strategic and front-line change management skills, which are often in short supply (see Chapters Five and Seven).

7 Where the organisation's existing knowledge and skills base is insufficient, then the use of external change agents to support implementation may be required but is unlikely to succeed unless there is a concerted effort to achieve a common language and values system, and shared meanings between the policy makers, the external facilitators and the front-line innovators, who will have differing, often incongruent, 'frames', cultures, concepts and vocabularies (see Chapter Seven).

For change leaders and managers: the use of design principles

Many of the above points for policy makers – especially Points 3-7 – apply also to change leaders and managers. Service innovation is a social and organisational process, which means that the introduction of innovation is predominantly a question of managing the social and organisational factors associated with that process rather than just the operational and technical ones. Below we detail – under seven headings – the main factors that we found to be relevant during our study of TCs and present them in the form of 'design principles' for service delivery innovation (Romme, 2003; van Aken, 2004, 2005a, 2005b).

Improvising skills for dealing with complexity, non-linearity and unpredictability

The innovation process is characterised by high levels of complexity, ambiguity, uncertainty and unpredictability (the 'innovation journey' is a contingent, non-linear, dynamic, responsive process), and no amount of planning and attempted control is ever likely to change or compensate for that. Therefore it is better, we believe, to take steps that allow change practitioners to work *with* these forces rather than incessantly wrestling to tame and get on top of them. The *management* of complexity (as opposed to the *resolution* of complexity) is thus core to the process and practice of innovation. Managers must learn to improvise effectively.

- Keep the portfolio of innovation initiatives to a manageable size; do not try to chase everything that appears (as, for example, did St Urban's and Robbleswade); informed opportunism is about making felicitous choices, not chasing every passing fad or initiative.
- Ensure that there is a concise business case for the innovation that is based on evidence about benefits and costs and has a clear vision, aims, financial forecasts and objectives (especially around capacity and demand estimates, skill mix, case mix and volume projections, key performance indicators, competitor analysis and the like). Over the three years of our study most TCs struggled and two completely failed because there were simply not enough patients; the business case had been built on hugely over-optimistic supply assumptions. Also be clear and upfront about motives, aspirations and intentions. This is your 'workable blueprint' (Van de Ven et al, 1999) or 'frozen ambitions' (van der Knaap, 2006). Being a relatively fixed point, it will help you navigate the innovation journey – especially helpful when (inevitably) you find yourselves blown off course or in stormy waters. Business and strategic planning of this kind needs to take precedence over detailed operational planning, which can itself become an increasing burden and source of anxiety when the reality begins to diverge, as it surely will, from the plan. Develop roomy, adaptive (as opposed to detailed, hard-wired) strategic plans – directional rather than detailed, but addressing *all* the key strategic 'choice points' for innovators (see Chapters Five and Seven).
- In this kind of unpredictable innovation environment, *prepare* as opposed to *plan*. People often plan because they are not properly equipped or prepared (in terms of skills, resources, shared vision, team effectiveness, motivation and direction); or put the other way

round, the more prepared (match fit) you and your team are, the less you may need to plan in huge amounts of detail.

- Do careful, systematic horizon scanning to pick up any distant clouds that might put future projections at risk. For TCs these included national developments such as Patient Choice, Payment by Results, changes to commissioning and involvement of the independent sector (see Chapter Four). Locally there were mergers, reorganisations, closures. None of these came completely out of the blue, and yet their possible impact had rarely been seriously thought about (see Chapter Five).

- Insist on flexible physical design to accommodate future innovation in both equipment and procedures (especially when there is the danger of building the wrong thing in haste). In the context of the pressurised planning that surrounded TCs, this concept of flexible design should have gone beyond physical buildings to embrace many other aspects of the innovation process, including the organisational and management dimensions (see Brindlesham, Chapter Five, for an example of effective flexibility).

- Build in flexible contingencies and formulate and rehearse multiple and explicit 'imagine if' scenarios.

- Avoid drowning in detail by focusing on key aspects of care/core measures/dashboards; measure only what is genuinely meaningful and helpful.

- Test flights for fledgling or early innovations can be useful. Encourage small-scale innovation experiments and develop and test various prototype solutions before spreading system-wide. Try to develop, dry run and test performance measurement, scheduling and planned booking, information and other systems in advance of going live. (The Department suggested leasing a TC facility to see how it works out but we are not aware of anyone actually having done that.)

- Do not concentrate on designing and planning to the detriment of implementation and trying out by doing – work from 'test flights' as opposed to trying to work it all out from the ground. Building to pilot and test, learning faster by failing early and giving permission to explore new behaviours are likely to be more productive than trying to theorise about and plan for everything in advance (Bate and Robert, 2007; Coughlan et al, 2007). (Note: To some extent this runs counter to what the Modernisation Agency was advocating in the way of TCs having detailed *operational* plans.) See Lakenfield (Chapter Six) for an example of effective enactment and enabling activity.

- Improvisation and improvisational behaviour warrant a special mention. There is growing evidence of extensive use and acceptance of improvisation in the management of change and innovation, not because it is fashionable or even necessarily creative but because it is the only way of coping with complexity and fast change and the flexible behaviour and spontaneous decision making they require (Crossan, 1997; Chelariu et al, 2002; Leybourne, 2007). Improvisation activity therefore needs to be built into the innovation process and also developed as a core competency by those involved.

- Finally we do not wish to give the impression that absolutely everything associated with the innovation process is unfathomable, unpredictable and unplannable. Much of it was, but a lot was not. It is important to differentiate between what is genuinely unknown and unknowable, and that which could be known if one knew how and where to look – the classic difference between uncertainty and ignorance. A good deal was not being (fore)seen simply because the planning techniques being used were insufficiently sensitive or accurate. In contrast to the rather crude intuitive planning and scheduling methods used by the TCs, there is the potential for even fairly conventional mathematical modelling and analytical tools to be deployed so as to reveal the many things that can actually be analysed and predicted, and hence to narrow the gap between what is currently known and could be known, such as predicting capacity requirements, optimising patient flows and bed capacity, managing variability, deciding whether an innovation will improve the efficiency and so on (Chapter Seven).

Creating 'enabling' structures and systems

It is worth the effort of establishing a specific organisational structure for the innovation process that can connect all the various roles together and provide functional coordination between them. The structure is not just to provide a mechanism of control and accountability during innovation and change but to enable new roles, behaviours, processes and patterns of behaviour to emerge, develop and ultimately intertwine to work as a system.

- Establish a core multidisciplinary, preferably multilevel, innovation team (a caucus of like-minded people) and take sufficient time to develop a shared aspiration and unity of purpose between its members. One of its activities should be to vigorously challenge the initial claims and assumptions contained in the business plan, which often turn out to be well wide of the actual mark.

- Clearly define all key roles and line responsibilities of those involved in the innovation process. Consider carefully the place of an innovation team leader ('modernisation lead') as part of the management framework.
- Establish complete transparency in staff recruitment and avoid favouritism (which was so damaging at Stanwick); try to anticipate where staff shortages are likely to be and where alternative arrangements may need to be put in place.
- Clarify and agree staff roles and specifications – including new gradings, terms and conditions – sooner rather than later. Get the structural basics sorted out early.
- Establish robust project management processes but avoid the heavy-handed administrative structures that take away the energy, enthusiasm and resilience of those involved until the innovation suffers death by project management.
- Do not organise innovative services in the abstract but tie the new structures into clinical processes, such as clear and agreed treatment protocols and care pathways.
- Be aware of the need to create new or extended roles that cross traditional boundaries and to challenge the logic of traditional structures, seeking not just alterations but real alternatives, such as schedulers, extended roles for therapists, advanced nurse practitioners (see, for instance, Lakenfield and Stanwick, Chapter Six).
- Create slack and carve out time for people to grow into these new roles and do not accept the view of innovation as overtime work on top of normal duties, an approach that can only be sustained for a limited time (see Northendon, Chapter Five).
- Establish sufficient linking and liaising roles (such as clinician managers, a service innovation team) and ensure they are effective vertically, horizontally (and diagonally!)
- Start early to build a marketing and communications strategy, structure and process. Innovation requires meticulous and continuous and unfailing communication, both internal and external.
- Staff turnover was often a problem, so endeavour to maintain continuity in key staff positions by recognising and rewarding people accordingly.
- Ensure there are suitable and clear overall targets (with key performance indicators) *and* incentives for performance.

- When establishing a new service, agree – and enforce – strict protocols for patient selection, and inform all relevant parties what these are.
- Ensure that adequate levels of information technology and support are available from the outset; for TCs this applied especially to booking systems (see, for instance, Pollhaven, Chapter Five).
- Attend to and put in place clinical and governance arrangements well in advance of opening a new facility.

Navigating the politics of innovation and securing stakeholder engagement

Innovations in health service delivery require collaboration between multiple professional and occupational groups and thus involve complex political challenges to unite their thinking and line them up behind the innovation. Antagonism between key players constantly threatens innovations (as happened at St Urban's, Pollhaven and Stanwick, among others) and therefore needs constant attention by building and maintaining the (highly fragile) 'negotiated order'.

- Engage, inform and involve the senior executive team, board and other senior people from the outset – and keep them involved.
- Clarify relationships and interdependencies between units, departments and the wider organisation; resist the natural drift into adversarial relationships, derogatory stereotypes and damaging them and us/win–lose dynamics (see Chapters Three and Five).
- Trust needs a special mention in this category: this research has shown repeatedly that once trust has broken down or been violated (especially between a healthcare provider and its community partners) the success of the innovation will be in serious jeopardy (for example, St Urban's, Robbleswade and Northendon).
- Align the innovation strategy to wider organisational strategies; ensure it fits in with local and regional development plans and avoid surprises for any of the key stakeholders (see St Urban's, Chapters Two and Five). Take care with the timing of your interventions.
- Address the things that motivate the key actors. Be aware of the incentives based on quantity, quality and kudos (see Chapter Three) and how they interact. Craft the case to suit and connect with their local agendas, ideals and concerns (examples might include efficiency and quality, hospital regeneration, improved working life – things that managers, clinicians and patients would see as the benefits or relative advantages); tap into the 'frames' of the powerful groups,

the opportunists, idealists, pragmatists and sceptics (see Chapters Three and Seven). Listen to the sceptics; they are often voicing the concerns of the silent majority and can help reveal the barriers to change; deal with opponents and adversaries by including them in the innovation process – leaving them out is only likely to increase the bickering, hostility or opposition (see, for example, Brindlesham, Pollhaven, St Urban's and Stanwick, Chapters Two and Five).

- Incentives and rewards are still among the most powerful ways of getting innovation adopted; these can be financial or non-financial.
- Find local innovation champions and leaders and empower them to take responsibility for getting their particular professional colleagues on board – using the principle that like recruits like (see, for instance, Lakenfield, Chapter Six).
- Develop new care pathways and models of care *with* those who are supposed to be adopting and following them; avoid imposition.
- Look for catalytic and 'piggy-back' events for promoting the innovation and winning the support from internal and external stakeholders. (The very act of bidding for a TC as a way of moving day care up the agenda was a very good example of this – see Chapters Two and Three.)

Building the innovation network

Organisational innovations like a new TC are not so much a technical exercise as a social, community and network-building enterprise, depending for their outcome on the assistance and support of a wide range of people.

- Do not try to foist your innovation on the wider health community: make dialogue and dense face-to-face interaction an external as well as internal feature of the innovation process. (Innovation is about building relationships, especially trust – see above.)
- Build and nurture close and constructive relationships with local health community partners, including GPs, and direct links with community groups through meetings and consultation exercises. Search out possible strategic partnerships and alliances, including, if appropriate, the independent sector (as at Brindlesham).
- Link with specialist external groups and make use of the expertise, protection and networking capacity of agencies set up for that purpose (as TCs did with NHS Elect, see Chapters Three and Four) or other more informal communities of practice.

- Develop and nurture communities of practice (Wenger, 1998, Wenger et al, 2002) that involve multiple stakeholders, both at managerial and clinical levels (see Chapter Seven). These – especially if they include or have close links to, respected opinion leaders – may generate more effective ways to share ideas and build on collective experience, develop working knowledge and skills, provide solutions to problems, increase feelings of ownership and facilitate sustainability resulting in enhanced job satisfaction and better working environments, but they can also create barriers for those who are not part of them, so beware communities of practice becoming cliques (le May, 2009).

Creating a learning process

Innovation and change processes are also learning processes – no learning, no change. 'Learning' in this regard needs to address not only knowledge and skills but also awareness-raising and development.

- Treat the innovation as a continual individual and group learning and development opportunity. Seek opportunities to embed a questioning culture into the innovation process. For example, set out systematically to treat setbacks as opportunities for learning (not blame).
- Use communities of practice to develop learning about the innovation and change processes (le May, 2009).
- Create from the start a parallel formative evaluation alongside the innovation process, so that events and experiences can be learned from and a continuous reflection/improvement/refinement cycle established. This might even include internal and external (action) research about the innovation process.
- Use this and other opportunities to raise awareness about the process of innovation and change and to challenge assumptions about its nature, for example whether patients – and clinicians! – would be prepared to travel to the new facility (Pollhaven).
- Identify any skills gaps early on and address these by way of dedicated training and development programmes. Such programmes will cover skills training but also behavioural, attitudinal and mindset issues (see, for example, Lakenfield, Stanwick and Robbleswade).
- Look for and take advantage of any free expertise in the system. Ensure, for example, that members of the core team attend specialist workshops, conferences and other learning events; visit other sites

and belong to – or establish – relevant communities of practice across sites.

- Obtain regular feedback on improvements (or not) in both patient and staff experience; establish a network of trusted informants.
- Conduct a summative ('how did we do?'/'learning for judgement') evaluation at discrete stages of and/or at the end of the project to capture the lessons retrospectively and build them into a set of design principles ('if you want to achieve outcome Y in situation S, we found that something like X helped') for future innovation. All-staff reflective review (away) days for all involved staff may help to achieve this.
- Be continually on the lookout for possible unintended consequences or spin-offs from the innovation (positive and negative – for example, resentment and hostility from the host organisation) and learn from them so as to help those running the new facility to respond appropriately.

Changing behaviour and culture

Innovation is about changing mindsets and behaviours so that people think and do things differently. We found that it was all too easy for an innovation attempt to become mired in the traditional patterns of activity and to end up more of a replication than an innovation. All the sites experienced the brake effects of the existing trust culture, but some were ultimately more successful in overcoming them than others (see Chapters Five and Six).

- Try to develop an awareness of the inhibiting brake effects of existing cultural practices and traditional mindsets; constantly challenge the apparent common sense in which culture meanings are wrapped. Resist attempts to normalise and reincorporate the innovation back into the normal frame of 'the way we do things around here'. It may be hard to see when such cultural effects are happening, and because 'the fish is the last to see the water', it helps to look at the organisational culture from outside, including, for example, asking patients and carers to reflect back how they see and experience the culture. It also helps to value and reward unconventional thinking.
- Focus on building a distinct identity for the innovation that patients and staff can relate to and value, including perhaps an image that 'badges' and brands the innovation and establishes its unique selling point and attracts attention and support in the wider field. For example, the decision whether to call a TC a TC or not was

important (labels did matter), as was the question of whether staff loyalties should be primarily to the TC or to the wider trust.

- Also concentrate on developing a strong and supportive ethic or ethos around the innovation. Northendon, for example, stressed openness, honesty, treating staff and patients with dignity and respect. Others focused on listening and encouraging feedback; or giving treatment based on the 'wellness' rather than 'illness' model; or guaranteeing continuity of care. But avoid empty rhetoric that merely generates cynicism when it is not matched by actions.
- Opening ceremonies and official launch events were a useful symbol of the importance being attached to the innovation. Other symbols included recognition for service excellence, for example, TC nurse of the year award, Chair's award.
- Reward and celebrate achievements, including good 'citizenship' behaviours (for example, support activities that go beyond the normal call of duty).
- Concentrate on building a strong team-based, entrepreneurial 'can do' mentality that was evident in a number of TCs (see Chapter Six) and reflects the values of 'positive organisational scholarship' (see Chapter Seven, note 5).

Leadership

- Look for emergent and rising leaders who want to champion the innovation, rather than 'the usual suspects'.
- Adopt as far as possible a 'help it happen' as opposed to 'make it happen' or 'let it happen' approach (see Figure 7.2).
- Move from a rule-based to an incentive-based form of leadership: 'pull' rather than 'push' leadership.
- Leaders need to be aware of the importance of 'framing to fit' – telling the 'innovation story' in a way that appeals to and resonates with the values, sentiments and goals of key audiences (see Chapter Seven, *Differing Frames*).
- Participation and inclusion are the watchwords of leadership for this form of innovation despite the natural temptation to keep one's cards to one's chest and to exclude external parties from decision making (as happened, for instance, at St Urban's).
- Establish a leadership system or process that is based on professional leadership lines, but avoids interprofessional sectarianism. Depending on the nature of the innovation, clinical leaders may prove to be the first among equals for the innovation, as happened in some TCs, and this needs to be carefully managed.

Implications for research

In this final section we address the implications of our study for future research, noting that 'the empirical literature on the implementation of service innovations in healthcare is currently extremely sparse' (Greenhalgh et al, 2005, p 18).

- Research is needed on the appropriate balance between centrally generated innovations and those that are generated locally and disseminated laterally. In the NHS, as in most health services, the continual swing of the pendulum between centrist, top-down and devolved, bottom-up management should provide useful natural experiments.
- Given that the standing of the eight sample TCs was in general better at the time of writing (2010) than it was in 2006 at the end of our three years of fieldwork, there may be an argument for longer-term studies of health service organisational innovation, to investigate how and why changes develop over the long run.
- Work is needed to help develop and evaluate the concept and use of 'design principles' in facilitating successful innovation, perhaps using an action research or formative evaluation design to explore the place of design principles for organisational innovation at the local level.
- The nature and place of positive organisational scholarship (see Chapter Seven, note 5) as a means of fostering a more receptive environment for organisational innovation might be further explored empirically.
- We need to understand more about how middle managers and front-line staff in health service organisational innovations such as TCs make sense of and therefore contribute to change outcomes in different contexts.[1] Relatedly, more work is needed to understand how the inevitable contests and negotiations of meaning in multilevel and multidisciplinary organisations ('frames' – see Chapter Seven) can be more successfully reconciled. In particular, qualitative research on innovation needs to be alert to the ways in which the perceptions of those working on an innovation can both under- and overplay the changes they engender or experience ('the glass half full' – see Chapter Six).
- A highly relevant methodological question, which we have struggled with in a number of other organisational studies in the NHS, is how researchers can best handle the problem of studying an organisational entity that is subject to a range of – sometimes incompatible – meanings held by key players. This problem is heightened when

the research sponsors subscribe to just one of those conflicting perceptions and/or expect researchers to measure success against targets and criteria defined by policy makers but when these are being imperceptibly, perhaps deceptively, transformed by front-line managers and staff (Pope et al, 2007).

• A study is needed to explore the barriers and opportunities for using theoretical planning exercises and operational research as part of introducing organisational innovations. In particular what might better facilitate the influence of such evidence on service delivery and organisation within health services? How might modellers and operational researchers dispel the problem currently affecting much of their work (often referred to as the 'Cassandra complex', recalling the Trojan prophetess who was condemned by a piqued god always to be ignored, even when she correctly predicted the wooden horse).[2]

• What are the sources of evidence that decision makers draw on when making the decision to innovate, and how are these played out in the negotiations and debates that precede the decision and subsequently shape its journey? In particular, how do political and power relations and organisational roles impact on this process (Gabbay et al, 2003)? In the terms developed by Gabbay and le May (2011), how do colleagues share and modify their 'knowledge-in-practice-in-context' about innovations as modifications to their collective internalised guidelines for practice (their 'mindlines')?

Notes

[1] This research recommendation also builds on the conclusions of Balogun and Johnson's (2005) study.

[2] Of relevance to both of these questions is the work of MASHnet, funded by the Engineering and Physical Sciences Research Council. (For further information see MASHnet, 2006, at http://mashnet.info/.)

Early definitions of a treatment centre

Treatment centres (TCs) were intended to deliver high volumes of high quality care using modern, efficient methods based on well-designed care-pathways. The key was separating elective from emergency care so that TCs could concentrate on delivering booked services according to planned protocols with the additional benefit of routinely offering patients choice and convenience. To achieve these aims, there was a guiding expectation that novel patient pathways would be planned that did not necessarily treat conventional departmental or professional boundaries as sacrosanct. The new model of care was expected to be innovative in focusing on the needs of patients rather than of the organisation and, where possible, providing a one-stop shop where the provision of diagnostic *and* treatment services improved both the efficiency of the service and the experience of the patient.

These defining characteristics of TCs were frequently reiterated in Department of Health and NHS material. Such sources also frequently repeated the point that there was no single model for a TC, whether run by the NHS or the private sector. Rather than a single model for all circumstances, TCs could be anywhere on a continuum from relatively simple primary care-based developments through traditional day case units to full blown elective 'factories' For example:

> The term Diagnostic and Treatment Centres encompasses a wide range of healthcare activities and types of facility. (SDC Consulting, 2001)

> Treatment Centres will vary in the types of services they offer depending on the local demand for health services. (Treatment Centres FAQ, originally at http://dh.gov. uk/PolicyAndGuidance/OrganisationPolicy, last accessed September 2006.)

> For the NHS, DTCs [Diagnostic and Treatment Centres] offer an opportunity to adopt best practice and increase short term capacity through new ways of working. There

> is not one prescribed model for a DTC; for example it could be on NHS property or in a shopping centre. There are no set ideas on structure as long as the DTC is fit for purpose. Trusts may even want to consider leasing a facility and learning from how this works before building a tailor-made DTC. (Ken Anderson of the Department of Health's independent sector TC team, quoted in Architects for Health, 2003)

The NHS Modernisation Agency, which had been set up to oversee and guide the modernising of the NHS (see Chapter Four) had the task of coordinating a collaborative programme to support these developments in TCs. By the time our study began in 2003, the Modernisation Agency's website gave the following as a description of the core characteristics (*the desiderata*) of a TC:

> The goal of a Treatment Centre is to deliver high quality, cost effective scheduled diagnostic and/or treatment services that optimise service efficiency and clinical outcomes and maximise patient satisfaction.
>
> The defining characteristics of a Treatment Centre are that
>
> (1) it embodies throughout its life the very best and most forward thinking practice in the design and delivery of the services it provides
> (2) it delivers a high volume of activity in a pre-defined range of routine treatments and/or diagnostics
> (3) it delivers scheduled care that is not affected by demand for, or provision of, unscheduled care either on the same site or elsewhere
> (4) its services are streamlined and modern, using defined patient pathways
> (5) its services are planned and booked, with an emphasis on patient choice and convenience together with organisational ability to deliver
> (6) it has a clear and trusted identity that is valued by its patients and by its other stakeholders
> (7) it provides a high quality, positive patient experience
> (8) it creates a positive environment that enhances the working lives of the people who work in it
> (9) it adds significantly to the capacity of the NHS to treat its patients successfully. (NHS Modernisation Agency, 2003c)

The study design and methods

Sampling and site access

We used a multi-method case study design (Eisenhardt, 1989; Yin, 1994, 2003). We selected eight case study sites, using the preliminary information that we had gathered in preparation for the proposal. The selection of sites was also informed by meetings with the director and members of the NHS Modernisation Agency team responsible for the treatment centre (TC) programme. The sampling was intended to ensure that the case study sites provided a broad representation of the range of TCs either existing or in development as at March 2003 when the research began.

The selection characteristics that we considered were:

- geographical (for example, urban/rural);
- type of host trust;
- organisational (for example, integral or separate from host trust; NHS 'star rating' of host trust; likelihood of foundation hospital status);
- intended case mix (such as single or multiple specialty, routine or more complex cases);
- the stage of development (from those that were already open, through to those in the early planning stage);
- scale (as measured in terms of planned numbers of patients);
- new/purpose-built or not;
- degree of private sector involvement;
- commissioning model (such as whether reliant on multiple or single commissioners).

Ethical approval for the study was sought from a Multi-centre Research Ethics Committee in January 2003, and full approval was granted on 14 April 2003 (MREC/03/07). Management approval for the study from the relevant NHS trust chief executive or TC director in each of the sites was then obtained.

All but one of our original choices agreed to be case study sites (see Table A2.1). The sites were given an information sheet about the study. When they had accepted, a local 'site representative' was appointed from among the senior staff associated with the TC. With the help of this person, key initial informants in each site were selected for interview, based on their roles and involvement with the TC.

The sites selected ranged from relatively small initiatives (a single ward, Phase I of Lakenfield) to much larger enterprises including centres that operated essentially as a mini-hospital (Ruckworth and Robbleswade). Some were new purpose-built facilities (Robbleswade, Stanwick, Northendon, Pollhaven and Phase II of Lakenfield), some were refurbishments of facilities within the host organisation – usually a hospital (Brindlesham and St Urban's) – and one (Ruckworth) was a separate leased building. The earliest date of opening was Lakenfield in 2000 with the latest (the same hospital's Phase II) originally due to open in 2007/08, finally opening in 2010. The sites varied in terms of activity or scale as measured by the approximate number of patients intended to be treated per annum when the TC was fully operational (measured in 'finished consultant episodes'). Ruckworth and Robbleswade were expected to have the highest activity, over double that of the smaller sites like Stanwick and Pollhaven. All the sites eventually selected were based in acute trusts and perhaps because of this most were in urban settings, although the geographical locations covered included city centres and towns near more rural and/or seaside areas. Robbleswade had major private sector involvement in the building work but was an NHS facility. The organisational status of the sites included trusts with between 0-3 stars and one was granted foundation hospital status during the course of the study; others were also in various stages of planning to do so.

The fieldwork, described more fully below, was undertaken over two-and-a-half years between mid-2003 and early 2006. It principally entailed organisationally focused interviews with key informants who were either involved in the design and delivery of the TC or in receipt of its services, direct observation of the TC's workings (such as site development, TC meetings and educational events) and documentary review (including business plans, board minutes and annual reports). In addition, to contextualise our case study work, we undertook a comprehensive literature review of published and grey literature, some of which is reported in Chapter One, and kept abreast of relevant national policy changes (see Chapter Four).

Fieldwork

We carried out the interviews in two phases, the first focusing on the internal organisation of the TC and its host trust, the second on members of the local health economy such as representatives of relevant primary care trusts (PCTs), strategic health authorities (SHAs) and neighbouring trusts. We used a snowball sampling technique in both phases, starting in phase one with the initial key players (such as the chief executive of the host trust and the TC manager or core team members) as identified by our site representatives. These early interviewees were asked to recommend other significant informants and so on until, again with the help of the site representative, we considered the sample to be complete across all the relevant parts of the system. We also consulted key personnel at the Modernisation Agency and several of our sites were members of NHS Elect, which led us to interview senior staff from this organisation as part of the second phase of our fieldwork (see Chapter Four).

Table A2.1: The sites

Site	Open	Planned cases/ year*	Physical relation to host hospital
Ruckworth	2002	7,000	Separate site, stand-alone
Lakenfield	2003 2010	4,000	a) Continuation of pilot on a ward in the host trust, first opened in 2000 b) New build, linked by bridge
Robbleswade	2005	7,000	New build extension to a recently built hospital
Stanwick	2004	3,000	New build extension to existing old hospital
Brindlesham	2003	5,000	Refurbishment of existing building on host site
St Urban's	2002	4,000	Major refurbishment of private patients' wing in host hospital trust
Northendon	2003	5,000	New build extension to host hospital
Pollhaven	2004	3,000	New build extension to existing hospital

Note: * to nearest thousand.

Interviews were semi-structured and were nearly all audio-recorded and transcribed. Most were face to face, sometimes with more than one interviewee at the same time. Where necessary, in a minority of instances, the interviews were done by telephone. We used a set of interview prompts to guide our approach throughout to ensure consistency between members of the research team.

We carried out 201 interviews in all, across a range of categories of interviewees, who may have been interviewed between one and five times (see Table A2.2).

Table A2.2: The interviewees

Category of interviewee	Number interviewed in each category
Host trust	
Chief executive	5
Senior trust managers	30
TC project coordinators	9
TC non-clinical managers	24
TC clinical leads	32
TC clinical managers	17
Other clinical specialists	7
Other support specialists	6
External stakeholders	
PCT chief executive	5
PCT senior managers	9
SHA senior managers	13
Other hospital managers	3
Others miscellaneous managers	6
Modernisation Agency links to TCs	3

At most sites we also undertook opportunistic non-participant observation of:

- decision-making interactions (such as formal and informal networking within the TCs: project management meetings, clinical pathways design groups, staff 'away days' and training events run by external consultants; discussions between TCs and their parent organisation: trust board meetings which focused on TC-related topics such as capacity planning, case mix and complaints; discussions between the TCs and service users: patient involvement and open days; meetings between TC members at the Modernisation Agency's TC learning events); and

- the processes of care and the physical environment of the TCs (such as guided tours of facilities/patient pathways, visits to building site to view construction; staff open days).

We carried out documentary analysis of, for example, business plans; minutes from internal TC team meetings, trust board meetings and the like; protocols and guidelines; press cuttings; key sources of information such as guidance for clinicians, websites and information sheets and booklets provided to patients and their carers. These analyses complemented the data gathered from the observation and interviews described above.

Patient interviews: because of the emerging emphasis of the study towards organisational and policy questions, and also because the NHS rules on ethical approval changed midway through the study, we did not interview patients.

Analysis

The qualitative research team iteratively shared and thematically analysed the data, building theory from the case studies along the lines described by Eisenhardt (1989):

- *analysing within-case* data, which involved for each site several detailed case study write-ups and presentations to the team;
- *searching for cross-case patterns*, for example selecting categories and then looking for between-case similarities and differences;
- *shaping propositions*, an iterative process in which we worked as a team to sharpen our constructs and definitions, building and re-examining the evidence to assess the constructs in each case; and where possible verifying and testing our emerging ideas – often during the interviews themselves – with those involved;
- *enfolding literature*: comparison of emergent concepts and hypotheses with the existing literature;
- *reaching closure*: deciding when 'theoretical saturation' was reached.

Once that stage had been reached, each member of the team produced 'site analyses' for the TCs they had been researching, which contained all the relevant material, extracted directly from the data and organised according to the main themes that had emerged. These analyses formed the basic material from which the research report was drafted by a team member, with all team members having a part in helping to shape and refine it. Before being released, the report was reviewed by anonymous external peer reviewers and also offered to senior managers at the case study sites for their reflections, comments and corrections, which were incorporated into the report produced by the National Institute for Health Research Service Delivery and Organisation (NIHR SDO) Programme. This book, written four years later, is the product of editing that report.

Note

[1] Two of the original research team (Bate and Robert) were involved in an interview-based survey of *all* the early NHS TCs. Further details of this work, funded by the NHS Modernisation Agency, can be obtained from the authors.

References

Anonymous (2003) 'Procure 21 cuts DTCs', *Contract Journal*, 4 September, p 1.

Architects for Health (2003) 'Summary of presentations and discussions', Conference on 'Diagnostic and Treatment Centres: the future of healthcare?', London: Architects for Health.

Augustine, S., Payne, R., Sencindiver, F. and Woodcock, S. (2005) 'Agile project management: steering from the edges', *Communications of the ACM*, vol 48, pp 85-9.

Balogun, J. and Johnson, G. (2005) 'From intended strategies to unintended outcomes: the impact of change recipient sensemaking', *Organization Studies*, vol 26, no 11, pp 1573-601.

Bartunek, J.M. and Moch, M.K. (1987) 'First order, second order, and third order change and organization development interventions: a cognitive approach', *The Journal of Applied Behavioral Science*, vol 23, pp 483-500.

Bate, S.P. and Robert, G. (2003) 'Where next for policy evaluation? Insights from researching NHS modernisation', *Policy & Politics*, vol 31, pp 237-51.

Bate, S.P. and Robert, G. (2005) 'Choice. More could mean less', *British Medical Journal*, vol 331, pp 1488-9.

Bate, S.P. and Robert, G. (2006) '"Build it and they will come" – or will they? Choice, policy paradoxes and NHS Treatment Centres', *Policy & Politics*, vol 34, pp 651-72.

Bate, S.P. and Robert, G. (2007) *Bringing user experience to health care improvement: The concepts, methods and practices of experience-based design*, Oxford: Radcliffe Publishing.

Bate, P., Robert, G., Gabbay, J., Gallivan S., Jit, M., Utley, M., le May, A., Pope, C. and Elston, M. (2006) *The development and implementation of NHS Treatment Centres as an organisational innovation*, London: NCCSDO (National Institute for Health Research Service Delivery and Organisation Programme) (National Co-ordinating Centre for NHS Service Delivery and Organisation) (*www.sdo.nihr.ac.uk/files/project/45-final-report.pdf*).

Beckhard, R. (1997) *Agent of change: My life, my practice*, San Francisco, CA: Jossey-Bass.

Bevan, H., Robert, G., Bate, S.P., Maher, L. and Wells, J. (2007) 'Using a design approach to assist large-scale organizational change: "ten high impact changes" to improve the National Health Service in England', *The Journal of Applied Behavioral Science*, vol 43, pp 135-52.

Black, A. (1999) 'High speed ahead', *Health Service Journal*, 10 June, Supplement: Special Report on Ambulatory Care, pp 1-4.

Blauner, R. (1964) *Alienation and freedom: The factory worker and his industry*, Chicago, IL: Chicago University Press.

Bowers, J., Jeffrey, S. and Mould, G. (2002) 'On defining ambulatory care in practice', *British Journal of Healthcare Management*, vol 8, pp 305-9.

Bright, D.S. and Cameron, K.S. (2009) 'Positive organizational change: what the field of positive organizational scholarship offers to OD practitioners', in W.J. Rothwell, R.L. Sullivan, J.M. Stavros and A. Sullivan (eds) *Practicing organizational development*, San Francisco, CA: Jossey-Bass, pp 397-410.

Brooks, I. and Bate, S.P. (1994) 'The problems affecting change within the British civil service: a cultural perspective', *British Journal of Management*, vol 5, pp 177-90.

Brunsson, N. (1982) 'The irrationality of action and action rationality: decisions, ideologies and organisational actions', *Journal of Management Studies*, vol 21, pp 29-44.

Bryman, A. (1984) 'Organisational studies and the concept of rationality', *Journal of Management Studies*, vol 21, pp 391-408.

Burge, P., Devlin, N., Appleby, J., Rohr, C. and Grant, J. (2005) *London Patient Choice Project evaluation. A model of patients' choices of hospital from stated and revealed preference choice data*, Cambridge: RAND Corporation.

Cameron, K.S., Dutton, J.E. and Quinn, R.E. (eds) (2003) *Positive organisational scholarship. Foundations of a new discipline*, San Francisco, CA: Berrett-Koehler.

Carvel, J. (2005) 'Eye of a storm', *The Guardian*, 26 January.

Casalino, L.P. and Robinson, J.C. (2003) 'Alternative models of hospital–physician affiliation as the United States moves away from tight managed care', *Milbank Quarterly*, vol 81, pp 331-51.

Casalino, L.P., Pham, H. and Bazzoli, G. (2004) 'Growth of single-specialty medical groups', *Health Affairs*, vol 23, pp 82-90.

Champoux, J.E. (1996) *Organisational behaviour. Integrating individuals, groups and processes*, St Paul, MN: West Publishing.

Chelariu, C., Johnston, W.J. and Young, L. (2002) 'Learning to improvise, improvising to learn: a process of responding to complex environments', *Journal of Business Research*, vol 55, pp 141-7.

Cohen, M.D., March, J.G. and Olsen, J.P. (1972) 'A garbage can model of organizational choice', *Administrative Science Quarterly*, vol 17, pp 1-25.

Conner, D.R. (2006) *Managing at the speed of change: How resilient managers succeed and prosper where others fail*, London: Random House Publishing Group.

Coughlan, P., Fulton Suri, J. and Canales, K. (2007) 'Prototypes as design tools for behavioural and organisation change: a design-based approach to help organisations change work behaviours', *The Journal of Applied Behavioral Science*, vol 43, pp 122-34.

Crossan, M. (1997) 'Improvising to innovate', *Ivey Business Quarterly*, Autumn, pp 36-42.

Daft, R.L. (1995) *Organisational theory and design* (5th edn), St Paul, MN: West Publishing.

Damiani, M., Propper, C. and Dixon, J. (2005) 'Mapping choice in the NHS: cross sectional study of routinely collected data', *British Medical Journal*, vol 330, p 284.

Darzi, A. (2008) *High quality care for all: NHS Next Stage Review final report*, London: Department of Health.

De Lathouwer, C. (1999) 'Ambulatory surgery: an organisational and cultural revolution, a social and political challenge', *Ambulatory Surgery*, vol 7, pp 183-6.

DH (Department of Health) (2000a) *The NHS Plan: A plan for investment, a plan for reform*, Cm 4818-I, London: The Stationery Office.

DH (2000b) *For the benefit of patients*, London: The Stationery Office.

DH (2002a) *Shifting the balance of power: The next steps*, London: The Stationery Office.

DH (2002b) *Delivering The NHS Plan: Next steps on investment, next steps on reform*, Cm 5503, April, London: The Stationery Office.

DH (2002c) *Reforming financial flows: Introducing payment by results*, London: The Stationery Office.

DH (2002d) *Growing capacity: Independent sector Diagnosis and Treatment Centres*, December, London: The Stationery Office.

DH (2003a) *Building on the best: Choice, responsiveness and equity in the NHS*, London: The Stationery Office.

DH (2003b) 'Renaming of Diagnosis and Treatment Centres', Chief Executive Bulletin 190, October, pp 10-16 (www.dh.gov.uk/en/ Publicationsandstatistics/Bulletins).

DH (2004) *The NHS Improvement Plan: Putting people at the heart of public services*, London: The Stationery Office.

DH (2005a) *Treatment Centres: Delivering faster, quality care and choice for NHS patients*, London: The Stationery Office.

DH (2005b) *Health reform in England: Update and next steps*, London: The Stationery Office.

DH (2006a) *Independent sector Treatment Centres*, A report from Ken Anderson, Commercial Director, Department of Health to the Secretary of State for Health, 16 February.

DH (2006b) *The NHS in England: The operating framework for 2006/07*, London: The Stationery Office.

Donabedian, A. (2003) *An introduction to quality assurance in health care*, Oxford: Oxford University Press.

Donnelly, L. (2005) 'When F is for failure', *Health Service Journal*, 29 September, pp 14-15.

Durant, G.D. (1993) 'Expanding the scope of ambulatory surgery in the USA', *Ambulatory Surgery*, vol 1, pp 173-8.

Durant, G.D. and Battaglia, C.J. (1993) 'The growth of ambulatory surgery centers in the United States', *Ambulatory Surgery*, vol 1, pp 83-8.

Eisenhardt, K.M. (1989) 'Building theories from case study research', *Academy of Management Review*, vol 14, pp 532-50.

Evans, O. (2007) 'Wave three Treatment Centres axed', *Health Service Journal*, 2 August.

Exworthy, M., Berney, L. and Powell, M. (2002) 'How great expectations in Westminster may be dashed locally': the local implementation of national policy on health inequalities, *Policy & Politics*, vol 30, no 1, pp 79-96.

Exworthy, M. and Peckham, S. (2006) 'Access, choice and travel: implications for health policy', *Social Policy and Administration*, vol 40, pp 267-87.

Ferlie, E., Freeman, G., McDonnell, J., Petsoulas, C. and Rundle-Smith, S. (2006) 'Introducing choice in the public services: some supply-side issues', *Public Money and Management*, January, pp 63-72.

Fonseca, J. (2002) *Complexity and innovation in organizations*, Oxford: Routledge.

Gabbay, J. and le May, A. (2011) *Practice-based evidence for healthcare: Clinical mindlines*, London: Routledge.

Gabbay, J., le May, A., Jefferson, H., Webb, D., Lovelock, R., Powell, J. and Lathlean, J. (2003) 'A case study of knowledge management in multi-agency consumer-informed "communities of practice": implications for evidence-based policy development in health and social services', *Health. An Interdisciplinary Journal for the Social Study of Health, Illness and Medicine*, vol 7, pp 283-310.

Gallivan, S. (2005) 'Mathematical methods to assist with hospital operation and planning', *Clinical and Investigative Medicine*, vol 28, pp 326-30.

Gallivan, S. and Utley, M. (2002) *Cautionary tales related to Patient Choice systems*, London: Clinical Operational Research Unit Working Paper 638, University of London.

Gallivan, S. and Utley, M. (2005) 'Modelling admissions booking of elective in-patients into a Treatment Centre', *IMA Journal of Management Mathematics*, vol 16, pp 305-15.

Goffman, E. (1974) *Frame analysis*, Boston, MA: Northeastern University Press.

Greener, I. (2004) 'Health service organization in the UK: a political economy approach', *Public Administration*, vol 82, pp 657-76.

Greener, I. (2009) 'Towards a history of choice in UK health policy', *Sociology of Health and Illness*, vol 31, pp 309-24.

Greenhalgh, T., Robert, G., MacFarlane, F., Bate, S.P. and Kyriakidou, O. (2004) 'Diffusion of innovations in service organisations: systematic review and recommendations', *Milbank Quarterly*, vol 82, pp 581-629.

Greenhalgh, T., Robert, G., Bate, S.P., Macfarlane, F. and Kyriakidou, O. (2005) *Diffusion of innovations in health service organisations*, Oxford: Blackwells.

Halford, S. and Leonard, P. (2006) *Negotiating gendered identities at work: Place, space and time*, Basingstoke: Palgrave.

Ham, C. (2005) 'Money can't buy you satisfaction: US and UK health care: a special relationship?', *British Medical Journal*, vol 330, pp 597-9.

Ham, C., Kipping, R. and McLeod, H. (2003) 'Redesigning work processes in health care: lessons from the National Health Service', *Milbank Quarterly*, vol 81, pp 415-39.

Harrison, A. and Appleby, J. (2005) *The war on waiting for hospital treatment. What has Labour achieved and what challenges remain?*, London: The King's Fund.

Healthcare Commission (2007) *Independent sector Treatment Centres: A review of the quality of care*, London: Commission for Healthcare Audit and Inspection.

Health Services Journal (2005) 'ITC programme: a good idea badly implemented and full of policy contradictions', 20 January, p 3.

Helms-Mills, J. (2003) *Making sense of organisational change*, London: Routledge.

Hoque, K., Davis, S., and Humphreys, M. (2004) 'Freedom to do what you are told: senior management team autonomy in an NHS acute trust', *Public Administration*, vol 82, pp 355-75.

House, R., Rousseau, D. and Thomas-Hunt, M. (1995) 'The meso paradigm: a framework for the integration of micro and macro organisational behavior', *Research in Organizational Behavior*, vol 17, p 71.

House of Commons (2004) HC 98 House of Commons, Minutes of Evidence, taken before Health Committee Public Expenditure.

House of Commons Health Select Committee (2006) *Independent sector Treatment Centres. Fourth report of Session 2005-06, Volume I*, HC 934-I, London: The Stationery Office.

Jackson, C. (2002) 'Cutting into the market: rise of ambulatory surgery centers', *amednews.com*, 15 April.

Janis, I.L. (1972) *Victims of groupthink: A psychological study of foreign policy decisions and fiascoes*, Boston, MA: Houghton Mifflin Company.

Kanter, R.M. (1983) *The change masters: Innovations for productivity in the American corporation*, New York: Simon and Schuster.

Kanter, R.M. (1988) 'When a thousand flowers bloom: structural, collective, and social conditions for innovation in organisations', *Research in Organisational Behaviour*, vol 10, pp 169-211.

Kanter, R.M. (1989) *When giants learn to dance: Mastering the challenge of strategy, management, and careers in the 1990s*, New York: Simon and Schuster.

Kanter, R.M., Stein, B.A. and Jick, T.D. (1992) *The challenge of organizational change: How people experience it and manage it*, New York: The Free Press.

Le Grand, J. (2009) 'Choice and competition in publicly funded health care: Response to Hunter, Dixon and Saltman', *Health Economics, Policy and Law*, vol 4, pp 479-88.

le May, A. (ed) (2009) *Communities of practice in health and social care*, Oxford: Wiley Blackwell.

Leybourne, S. (2007) 'Culture and organisational innovation', *Organisation Development and Change Newsletter*, Winter, pp 11-13.

Lindblom, C. (1959) 'The science of muddling through', *Public Administration Review*, vol 19, pp 79-88.

McNulty, T. and Ferlie, E. (2002) *Re-engineering health care. The complexities of organisational transformation*, Oxford: Oxford University Press.

Marsh, I. (2006) *Sociology: Making sense of society* (3rd edn), Harlow: Pearson Education.

Meyers, P.W., Sivakumar, K. and Nakata, C. (1999) 'Implementation of industrial process innovations: factors, effects and marketing implications', *Journal of Product Innovation Management*, vol 16, pp 295-311.

Morgan, G. and Layton, A. (1999) 'All in the timing', *Health Service Journal*, 10 June, vol 12, Supplement.

Naylor, C. and Gregory, S. (2009) *Independent sector Treatment Centres*, London: The King's Fund.

NHS Elect (2004) *Welcome to NHS Elect*, London: NHS Elect.

NHS Estates (1996) *Ambulatory care and diagnostic centres: The experience of the Central Middlesex Hospital*, London: The Stationery Office.

NHS Estates (2001) *Diagnostic and Treatment Centres: ACAD, Central Middlesex Hospital. An evaluation*, London: The Stationery Office.

NHS Modernisation Agency (2003a) *NHS Treatment Centres: Core characteristics*, Leicester: NHS Modernisation Agency.

NHS Modernisation Agency (2003b) *Diagnosis and Treatment Centres: Lessons from the pioneers*, Leicester: NHS Modernisation Agency.

NHS Modernisation Agency (2003c) *Diagnostic and Treatment Centres: A new service model*, Leicester: NHS Modernisation Agency.

Pettigrew, A.M. (1985) *The awakening giant. Continuity and change in imperial chemical industries*, Oxford: Blackwell.

Pham, H.H., Devers, K.J., May, J.H. and Berenson, R. (2004) 'Financial pressures spur physician entrepreneurialism', *Health Affairs*, vol 23, pp 70–81.

Plumridge, N. (2008) 'Running out of steam?', *Public Finance*, 23 May.

Plsek, P., Bibby, J. and Whitby, E. (2007) 'Design rules grounded in the experience of managers: a system for organizational learning and pilot study of practical methods', *The Journal of Applied Behavioral Science*, vol 43, pp 153–70.

Pollock, A. (2009) 'Independent sector Treatment Centres: the first independent evaluation, a Scottish case study', *Journal of the Royal Society of Medicine*, vol 102, pp 278–86.

Poole, M.S. and Van de Ven, A.H. (2004) *Handbook of organizational change and innovation*, Oxford: Oxford University Press.

Pope, C., le May, A. and Gabbay, J. (2007) 'Chasing chameleons, chimeras and caterpillars: evaluating and organisational innovation in the National Health Service', in L. McKee, E. Ferlie and P. Hyde (eds) *Organizing and reorganizing: Power and change in health care organizations*, Basingstoke: Palgrave, pp 112–22.

Pope, C., le May, A. and Gabbay, J. (2010) 'People, place and innovation: how organisational culture and physical environment shaped the implementation of the NHS TC programme', in J. Braithwaite, P. Hyde and C. Pope (eds) *Culture and climate in healthcare organisations*, Basingstoke: Palgrave Macmillan, pp 60–69.

Pope, C., Robert, G., Bate, S.P., Gabbay, J. and le May, A. (2006) 'Lost in translation. Metamorphosis of meanings and discourse in organisational innovation and change processes: a multi-level case study', *Public Administration*, vol 84, pp 59–79.

Pressman, J.L. and Wildavsky, A. (1984) *Implementation: How great expectations in Washington are dashed in Oakland; Or, why it's amazing that federal programs work at all, this being a saga of the Economic Development Administration as told by two sympathetic observers who seek to build morals on a foundation of ruined hopes* (3rd edn), Berkeley, CA: University of California Press.

Puranam, P., Singh, H. and Zollo, M. (2006) 'Organising for innovation: managing the coordination–autonomy dilemma in technology acquisitions', *Academy of Management Journal*, vol 40, pp 263–80.

Quinn, B. (1980) *Strategies for change: Logical incrementalism*, Homewood, IL: Irwin.

Reed, W.A. and Kershner, B.A. (1993) 'The history of the Federated Ambulatory Surgery Association', *Ambulatory Surgery*, vol 1, pp 18–21.

Reid, J. (2005) 'Limits of the market, constraints of the state: an NHS fair to all of us and personal to each of us', Speech to Social Market Foundation, 31 January, London (www.smf.co.uk/site/smf/Members/vjohnson/jr).

Ricketts, B. (2003) *Choice, capacity and productivity: Creating a virtuous circle*, Leicester: NHS Modernisation Agency.

Romme, A.G.L. (2003) 'Making a difference: organization as design', *Organization Science*, vol 14, pp 559–73.

Sanderson, I. (2002) 'Evaluation, policy learning and evidence-based policy making', *Public Administration*, vol 80, pp 1–22.

SDC Consulting (2001) *Salford's Health Investment for Tomorrow: Model of care proposal*, Discussion Paper, Salford: Salford's Health Investment for Tomorrow.

Seo, M.-G., Putnam, L.L. and Bartunek, J.M. (2004) 'Dualities and tensions of planned organizational change', in M.S. Poole and A.H. Van de Ven (eds) *Handbook of organizational change and innovation*, Oxford: Oxford University Press, pp 73–107.

Sillince, J.A.A., Harindranath, G. and Harvey, C.E. (2001) 'Getting acceptance that radically new working practices are required: institutionalization of arguments about change within a healthcare organization', *Human Relations*, vol 54, pp 1421–54.

Snow, D.A., Rochford, E.B., Worden, S.K. and Benford, R.D. (1986) 'Frame alignment processes, microbilization and movement participation', *American Sociological Review*, vol 51, pp 464–81.

Steffes, B.C. (1999) 'An ambulatory surgery center and minimally invasive surgery: lessons from experience', *Seminars in Laparoscopic Surgery*, vol 6, pp 2–10.

Stevens, S. (2005) 'Opinion', *Health Services Journal*, 13 January, p 17.

Stoeckle, J. (1995) 'The citadel cannot hold: technologies go outside the hospital, patients and doctors too', *Milbank Quarterly*, vol 73, pp 3-17.

Thompson, L. (2003) 'NHS Treatment Centres', NatPact (National Primary and Care Trust) Annual Conference, London.

Timmins, N. (2003) 'NHS group offers fast-track surgery', *Financial Times*, 16 October.

Traynor, M. (1999) *Managerialism and nursing: Beyond oppression and profession*, London: Routledge.

Utley, M. and Gallivan, S. (2004) 'Evaluating the new Diagnosis and Treatment Centres in the UK', in M. Dlouhy (ed) *Modelling efficiency and quality in health care: The proceedings of the 29th Meeting of the European Working Group on Operational Research Applied to Health Services*, Prague, July 2003, pp 125-32.

Utley, M., Gallivan, S. and Jit, M. (2005) 'How to take variability into account when planning the capacity for a new hospital unit', in J. Vissers and R. Beech (eds) *Health operations management*, London: Routledge, pp 146-61.

Utley, M., Gallivan, S. and Jit, M. (2009) 'Application of a simple analytical model of capacity requirements', in M. Lubicz (ed) *Operational research applied to health services in action*, Wroclaw: Oficyna Wydawnicza Politechniki Wroclawskiej.

Utley, M., Jit, M. and Gallivan, S. (2008) 'Restructuring routine elective services to reduce overall capacity requirements within a local health economy', *Health Care Management Science*, vol 11, pp 240-7.

van Aken, J.E. (2004) 'Management research based on the paradigm of the design sciences: the quest for tested and grounded technological rules', *Journal of Management Studies*, vol 41, pp 219-46.

van Aken, J.E. (2005a) 'Valid knowledge for the professional design of large and complex design processes', *Design Studies*, vol 26, pp 379-404.

van Aken, J.E. (2005b) 'Management research as a design science: articulating the research products of Mode 2 knowledge production', *British Journal of Management*, vol 16, pp 19-36.

van der Knapp, P. (2006) 'Responsive evaluation and performance management. Overcoming the downsides of policy objectives and performance indicators', *Evaluation*, vol 12, pp 278-93.

Van de Ven, A.H., Polley, D.E., Garud, R. and Venkataraman, S. (1999) *The innovation journey*, Oxford: Oxford University Press.

Warren, K.F. (1974) 'Book review: Implementation: how great expectations in Washington are dashed in Oakland; Or, why it's amazing that federal programs...', *The Journal of Politics*, vol 36, pp 1090-1.

Weick, K.E. (1979) *The social psychology of organising*, Reading, MA: Addison–Wesley.

Weick, K.E. (2001) *Making sense of the organization*, Oxford, UK and Malden, MA: Blackwell Publishing Ltd.

Wenger, E. (1998) *Communities of practice: Learning, meaning and identity*, New York: Cambridge University Press.

Wenger, E., McDermott, R. and Snyder, W. (2002) *Cultivating communities of practice*, Cambridge, MA: Harvard Business School.

Yin, R.K. (1994) *Case study research: Design and methods*, London: Sage Publications.

Yin, R.K. (2003) *Case study research* (3rd edn), Thousand Oaks, CA: Sage Publications.

Index

Page references for notes are followed by n